Acupuncture Cure for Common Diseases

For over 3000 years, millions of people in China and elsewhere in Asia have relied on acupuncture to promote, restore, and maintain good health. In the recent times the world outside has also recognised Acupuncture as a complete system of health care. Its effectiveness has now been well documented by the medical and scientific community and its application extends far beyond chronic pain management or as an analgesic.

Central to the concept of acupuncture is the idea that human body is a self-healing dynamic whole, full of energy and vitality which is being constantly regenerated and rebalanced from within. Acupuncture seeks to enhance body's natural healing processes by redirecting or realigning this energy, called Qi (pronounced 'Chi').

This book by one of India's leading team of practitioners of acupuncture is a comprehensive effort to explain how acupuncture can help in preventing and treating a wide range of physical, psychological, and emotional problems — both common and serious — and many of which modern medicine may not be able to cure. It describes how acupuncture works, its efficacy, the different techniques, and how the use of modern scientific methods has made it amongst the safest and the most effective drugless therapies.

The Authors

Dr Raman Kapur is one of the few doctors who have successfully combined the practice of modern medicine with acupuncture. After an MBBS degree from Delhi University, he trained in acupuncture in Switzerland and Sri Lanka before starting his practice. Today he runs one of the most successful acupuncture clinics in Delhi. He is also a Senior Honorary Consultant in acupuncture at New Delhi's prestigious Sir Gangaram Hospital.

His research in clinical acupuncture and remarkable success rate in treating chronic diseases won him a gold medal at the 33rd World Congress of Complementary Medicine held in Taiwan in 1992. Author of two books: *A Guide to Acupuncture and Tissue Cleansing System* and *Soft Lasers in Medical Practice*, he conducts courses and seminars on Acupuncture, Laser Therapy, Sonopuncture, and *Su Jok* Acupuncture.

Dr Sunita Kapur, an MBBS from Lady Hardinge Medical College, Delhi University, earned her diploma in acupuncture from Hong Kong. A fellow of the Acupuncture Federation of Korea and China and of the International Laser Therapy Association, she is actively associated in the acupuncture clinic with her husband, Raman Kapur.

ACUPUNCTURE CURE FOR COMMON DISEASES

Dr Raman Kapur, MBBS, MD (Acu.)
Dr Sunita Kapur, MBBS

Orient Paperbacks
DELHI | MUMBAI | HYDERABAD

The information given in this book is general in nature and for guidance only. It is not a substitute for medical advice and the readers are urged to consult their doctor before taking decisions which are medical in nature.

ISBN : 978-81-222-0232-8

Acupuncture Cure for Common Diseases

Subject: Health & Fitness / Acupuncture

1st Published 1999
8th Printing 2016

Published by
Orient Paperbacks
(A division of Vision Books Pvt. Ltd.)
5A/8, Ansari Road, New Delhi-110 002
www.orientpaperbacks.com

Cover design by Vision Studio

Printed at Yash Printographics, Noida

Contents

Preface

When I graduated in medicine many years ago, I entered the profession full of hope that I would be able to relieve suffering wherever I went. Gradually, however, I came to realise that most of the patients who came to me were being given symptomatic treatment — treatment which made them feel better but could not cure or even arrest the progress of the disease.

This led me to reassess whether Western medicine, which I had spent long years studying, was really the answer to better health. A critical evaluation revealed that the manner in which it was practised made it more symptomatic than curative. While it undoubtedly had effective remedies for certain ailments, especially emergencies and acute bacterial infections, there were a vast number of chronic diseases for which it had no solutions. Over the years, I came across numerous instances where Western medicine not only failed to cure the ailment, but caused considerable damage to the patient. As a result intelligent people everywhere had started exploring and seeking safer, alternative forms of health care which did not involve treatment that was potentially dangerous. This is how I got interested in learning the science of acupuncture.

'Acupuncture' means to cure diseases by puncturing with a needle. The Chinese philosophy of health and healing postulates that it is the energy flow in every living being that is responsible for life. They call this energy *Qi*. In a person who is sick, the energy flow is obstructed and imbalanced. Acupuncture achieves its curative effect by clearing the obstruction in the flow of *Qi* and balancing the energy flow. Once this energy flow is restored to normal, the person becomes and stays healthy.

Research and exhaustive studies conducted on acupuncture have brought out various truths. Western medicine, though helpful in certain diseases, has definite side-effects, whereas acupuncture is safe, harmless, and without any side-effects. The classical acupuncture system involves the use of very fine, thin, stainless steel needles at specific points; the system is entirely painless. And for patients who are afraid of needles, children, and women, various needleless techniques are available. Another very effective microsystem of acupuncture is known as *Su Jok Acupuncture* which can be learnt even by a layman and utilised for treating day-to-day problems. *Su Jok Acupuncture* utilises only the points on the hands and feet to treat all diseases.

During my two decades of clinical experience, I have treated thousands of patients suffering from various ailments with remarkable results. These range from arthritic and back pains, frozen shoulder, bronchial asthma, headaches and migraine, epilepsy, stomach problems, including ulcers, to different cardiovascular diseases and various kinds of de-addictions.

In addition to the conditions mentioned above, it is important to remember that acupuncture is a complete medical science which can be utilised to treat almost all known diseases and disorders.

This book is primarily intended for the lay person and the non-medical reader who wishes to know more about this ancient, yet very effective system of health care. Any patient who wishes to undergo acupuncture treatment would also find it helpful.

DR RAMAN KAPUR

'The sheer weight of evidence demands that acupuncture be taken seriously as a clinical procedure of considerable stature.'

R.H. Bannerman, M.D.
reporting on the
1979 conference of WHO in
American Journal of Acupuncture, July, 1980

1

Acupuncture: The Chinese Tradition of Health and Healing

Acupuncture is the ancient Chinese art of healing and is, probably, more than 5,000 years old. It is believed that once a Chinese soldier developed a stiff and painful shoulder for which, in spite of his doctor's best efforts, he could get no relief. One day, during a battle, a miracle occurred. The soldier's leg was wounded by an arrow and, suddenly, his stiff and painful shoulder of many years, could move freely again without pain.

This set observant physicians thinking — was there a relationship between the arrow wound and the relief from pain experienced by the soldier? To probe this thought further the wise men of Chinese medicine started mapping different points on the human body which had possible similar healing effects. Over a period of time they discovered that there existed many points located near the nerve endings, which when stimulated, had therapeutic effects. Using sharpened fish bones, bamboo sticks, and stone needles (*bians*), to stimulate these points, they began to chart their healing effects on different parts and organs of the body. It was surmised that there existed some kind of links or channels in the human body which carried these healing effects. And thus began the art and science of acupuncture.

In course of time nearly 800 points and twelve channels were identified. Each point, the size of a pinhead, was named after its discoverer which, when stimulated, had a beneficial effect on various illnesses and problems.

It is not known what this ancient Chinese system of healing was then called. What we do know is that the English word 'acupuncture' is derived from two Latin words: *acus,* meaning 'needle', and *puncture* meaning 'to penetrate'.

Acupuncture: Down the Ages

Though acupuncture is usually associated with the Chinese, it is not entirely of Chinese origin. Research has revealed that it was practised by the Bantus of South Africa, by Eskimos, and in ancient Brazil. There are strong indications that some form of acupuncture was prevalent in ancient India and that it travelled through Nepal to China. It is quite likely that it was preserved there and later amalgamated into the Chinese body of traditional medicine.

Very much like the other ancient healing systems, acupuncture too grew, developed, and flourished over a long period of time. Its practice was taught by one generation to the next, with sons inheriting the tradition of healing from their fathers.

The first written account of acupuncture can be

traced to the *Shi Ji Historical Records, circa* 200 BC. This work tells of Bia Que, a doctor in the 4th century BC, who became famous for bringing a prince out of coma by using acupuncture techniques. Probably the most important source of knowledge about acupuncture in ancient China is the great classic of Chinese medicine, *Huang Di Nei Jing* (The Yellow Emperor's Classic of Internal Medicine), compiled between 300 and 100 BC. Drawing on the traditions and perspectives of great Chinese thinkers such as Confucious, Tao Zi, Meng Zi, and Zhuang Zi it remains, even today, the basic text on the theory and philosophy of Chinese medicine.

Set as a conversation between Huang To, the Yellow Emperor, and his minister Qi Bo and others, the *Huang Di Nei Jing* outlines the principles of natural law and the movements of life: *Yin* and *Yang* (passive and active energies); *Wu Xing* — the five elements: water, wood, fire, earth, and metal; the interrelationship between Heaven, Earth, and Man; *Zang-Fu*: the organ system comprising the 12 organs of the body; *Jing-Luo*: the meridian network; *Qi* and blood; and the causes of disease — their effects, diagnosis, and treatment. It outlines the basic principles and differentiation of syndromes, describes the nine kinds of needles and their uses, and emphasises preventive treatment. A rich source book, *Huang Di Nei Jing*, in combination with the many later texts that exist as commentaries and amplifications, is used by acupuncturists even today.

A description of twelve channels and their treatment with moxibustion* (described in chapter 11), is also

* A form of a heat therapy in which moxa, the dried leaves of the herb *Artemisia vulgaris,* are ignited and applied directly or indirectly to acupuncture points (also called acu-points) as a form of treatment.

found written on silk scrolls in tombs dating from the Han dynasty, *circa* 200 BC.

Around AD 200, Huang Fu Mi's classic work on acupuncture and moxibustion was written. It details the accurate location of 349 acupuncture points, and, 1,700 years later, was used as a reference for the important modern work *Essentials of Acupuncture* (People's Publishing House, Beijing, 1979), compiled by the major acupuncture colleges of China.

During the rule of the Tang dynasty (AD 618-907), medical academies were established and the practice of acupuncture got a further fillip. Around AD 1026, the *Classic of Bronze Man* was written — an illustrated guide, it depicted acupuncture points on two life-size bronze figures. This work was engraved on two stone tablets, more than two metres high and seven metres wide, and became a standard work.

The 17th century marked the beginning of the decline of acupuncture and herbalism in China. This coincided with the increasing influence of Western ideas in China. In 1822, a government decree actually banned the practice of acupuncture from the Imperial Medical College, because undressing (even for medical examination) was considered improper. In Republican China (1911-1947), the Kuomintang government tried to ban traditional medicine in 1929 but, faced with protests from traditional doctors, its attempts failed. However, acupuncture seems to have fared worse in cities than in the countryside at this time.

Acupuncture in Modern China

When the People's Republic of China was formed in 1949, many of the revolutionary leaders were determined to rid their country of all religion and superstition, and to many of them this also included Traditional Chinese Medicine. Others, although accepting the usefulness of Western medicine, felt that traditional methods should also be preserved. A story is told that while on the Long March (1932-1933) Chairman Mao became very ill, and his life was saved by traditional folk medicine. He thereafter became a convert to traditional forms of medicine, and instituted a series of research projects in the 1950s about the scientific validity of acupuncture.

In 1958, after thousands of tests, the members of the Central Committee were convinced that traditional medicine was effective, and the Western and the Traditional Chinese Medicine were given equal status in the People's Republic of China.

During the Cultural Revolution (1966-1967), following the persecution of surgeons and doctors practising Western medicine, Traditional Chinese Medicine was given new opportunities to develop. Hospitals and training centres for Traditional Chinese Medicine were established throughout China. Many new methods were experimented with. These included needle-embedding, point-injection therapy, electro-acupuncture, and analgesia.

As acupuncture became renowned for its effectiveness in pain control, it was introduced as anaesthesia during operations — a major step forward from its earlier primary use to control post-operative pain. Experimentation started with minor operations such as tooth extraction and was later extended to tonsillectomy, thyroidectomy, treatment of hernias, and finally to major operations on the limbs, thorax, and abdomen. Today acupuncture is used extensively, both for treating serious hospitalized patients as well as in the OPD (Out Patient Departments), and for treating acute as well as chronic cases.

The widespread use of acupuncture in China caught the Western imagination but, unfortunately, also led to the misconception that its effectiveness was limited only to pain control and anaesthesia.

China opened her doors once more to the world in the 1970s and three-month advanced courses in acupuncture, promoted by the World Health Organization, were started in major cities such as Beijing, Guang Zhon, Naijing, and Shanghai for foreign students. In China, a complete training in Traditional Chinese Medicine entails five years of study.

The status of acupuncture in many far eastern countries, such as Japan, Korea, Malaysia, and India is similar to that in China. It is used not only for pain control but also for treating a wide variety of conditions, including asthma, ulcers, high blood pressure, and angina.

Acupuncture: Beyond the Bamboo Curtain

Acupuncture first reached the attention of the West in the second half of the seventeenth century. The first European writer to mention the subject was a Dane, Jacob de Bondt, who was surgeon-general to the Dutch East India Company at Batavia. A more detailed account of the technique was given by another Dutchman, Willem ten Rhijne, who was a physician in the service of the Dutch East India Company. A number of other authors wrote accounts of acupuncture during the seventeenth century, and gradually a clearer picture began to appear. By the end of the century, it seems, acupuncture of a sort, and also moxibustion, were being practised in parts of Western Europe.

In the early eighteenth century clinical interest in these techniques (acupuncture and moxibustion) declined, though they still attracted scientific comment and several commentaries were written.

During the first half of the nineteenth century interest in acupuncture and moxibustion revived, consisting, however, of simply needling the painful area. Although some information about the channels and pulse diagnosis had reached Western countries, this made little impression on most Western doctors. The first book on acupuncture was written by L.V.J. Berlioz in France in 1816. He reported excellent results in treating rheumatism, arthritis, and stiff muscles and joints.

To a limited extent, acupuncture was used as a form of treatment in Germany. In England the first important advocate was J.M. Churchill, who published two books on acupuncture in 1821 and 1828, describing the success of acupuncture in treating musculoskeletal disorders (rheumatism, sciatica, back pain, and so on) and dropsy.

By the mid-nineteenth century, Leeds Infirmary in England had become a major acupuncture centre and the practice of acupuncture had reached North America. Soon, however, Western interest in acupuncture waned again, obviously indicating that its scientific basis was not acceptable enough.

In the early part of the twentieth century the French writer Soulie de Morant wrote some books on acupuncture, based on Chinese sources and Vietnamese and Japanese influences. However, it was only when President Nixon visited China in 1972 that acupuncture actually came to the attention of the main body of the Western medical profession. The fact that Chinese surgeons were performing operations using acupuncture instead of conventional anaesthesia to prevent pain, aroused considerable interest among doctors of modern medicine. A number of researchers undertook studies to try to find out how acupuncture analgesia (rather than anaesthesia, for the patients remained conscious throughout) worked.

Meanwhile, a surprising discovery was made in the West. It was found that the body produced opium-like substances — endorphins and enkephalins — whose properties included the suppression of pain. Experiments demonstrated that needling the acu-points caused the release of these substances into the blood. In 1982 British scientists, Melzack and Wall, introduced a theory about how pain impulses were transmitted in the nervous system. This too seemed to have some relevance to acupuncture.

These developments led to increased interest in acupuncture amongst the scientific and medical community, many of whom tried out acupuncture in practice and found that it worked.

On the whole, however, Western doctors did not approach the subject from a traditional point of view but instead tried to reinterpret the phenomenon within the framework of modern scientific understanding of how the human body works.

The Scientific Evidence

In order to access correctly and scientifically the effectiveness of acupuncture as a safe and inexpensive system of health care, the scientific community has been strongly advocating that it undergo the same kind of clinical tests and trials as accepted in the Western medicine.

Amongst the many research projects, the 1980 study undertaken at the University of California Los Angeles (UCLA), USA, is worth mentioning. The study was published in 1980 in the medical publication *Pain*. It concluded:

> 'Acupuncture therapy, when properly administered, is an extremely safe and effective procedure which may be indicated for the treatment of certain chronic pain problems .... Finally we recommend that its application for the treatment of pain be considered an accepted procedure, and no longer "experimental".'

The researchers also pointed out that their results, although positive, did not demonstrate the full potential of acupuncture because the requirements of the research controls prevented the full use of acupuncture techniques.

Another line of research was that conducted by the University of Pennsylvania School of Veterinary Medicine, USA, into the effects of acupuncture in the treatment of animals. This was particularly interesting in that it ruled out the commonly held belief that the effectiveness of acupuncture treatment depended on belief or the placebo effect. In fact this large weight of veterinary research helped convince the courts in Southern Texas that acupuncture does in fact work. The US District court of Southern Texas in July 1980 (quoted in *The Journal of Traditional Acupuncture Vol. VI No. 2*) when considering the status of acupuncture stated:

> 'Acupuncture has been practised for 2,000 to 5,000 years. It is no more experimental as a mode of treatment than is the Chinese language as a mode of communication. What is experimental is not acupuncture, but Westerners' understanding of it and their ability to utilize it properly.'

Another significant project to study the effects of acupuncture on patients suffering from chronic breathlessness took place at the Churchill Hospital, Oxford, England, in 1986. It was conducted by a Chinese doctor, using traditional methods of diagnosis and treatment with traditional acupuncture techniques.

Dr Chen, from the Friendship Hospital in Beijing, treated twenty-four patients with chronic obstructive pulmonary disease. This particular disease was chosen by the Western doctors monitoring the project because it is fairly straightforward to measure results.

Dr Chen treated the patients individually, according to their particular presenting patterns of disease. Twelve patients received 'real' treatment, while twelve received placebo treatment (although only two out of the twelve guessed that their treatment was any different).

The results were remarkable. Virtually all the patients receiving the 'real' treatment, showed improvement, particularly in their ability to perform physical tasks without becoming breathless. To all these patients the medical profession could offer no further help.

The project received serious attention by the medical community and was reported in *The Lancet* and in many of the British newspapers.

Thus, despite claims by both the American and British Medical Associations that acupuncture has not been proven to be an effective method of treatment, the increasing demand for acupuncture in the West really speaks for itself.

Acupuncture in India

Several historical records show that acupuncture was practised in ancient India. Many Chinese travellers who came to India and wrote extensively about the local treatment practices mention vedic therapeutic methods of needling. It has been said that ayurvedic texts contained acupuncture principles but the practice was discontinued due to the then unfavourable circumstances in India. Some of the Indian erudites even stated that people learnt acupuncture from Indian experts in Takshashila University (*circa* 100 BC).

Researchers have reported the mention of both acupuncture and Ayurveda in the ancient Buddhist texts which were used to teach Tibetans. Buddha was reportedly responsible for writing various texts on Indian medicine, which are jealously guarded by the Tibetan Buddhists today. Four *shastras* or texts were written by Buddha, of which the fourth *shastra* dealt with acupuncture, moxibustion, surgery, and also mentions that Tibet received acupuncture and medicine from India.

During the 6th century, through the process of cultural exchange between China and other countries, acupuncture and moxibustion were disseminated to south-east Asia and India. Miyun from Dun Huang of Gansu province is said to have introduced the therapeutic methods and prescriptions of Hua Tuo, the great man of Traditional Chinese Medicine and acupuncture to India. But reports regarding its subsequent practice or acceptance in India are obscure.

It was only in the 1950s that interest in acupuncture was regenerated in India through the pioneering role of Dr Bijoy Kumar Basu. Dr Basu was a member of the historic Indian Medical Mission to China (1938-1942). It is interesting to note that though he was a student of Western medicine, he made sincere attempts to develop this oriental healing art in his motherland. He realized the inherent values of acupuncture and laid stress on acupuncture training for both health workers and qualified doctors. It was the concept of the 'barefoot doctor' in China and its success that made him continously inspire and actively guide medicos and health workers of different social service organizations like the Peoples' Relief Committee and Dr Dwarakanath Kotnis Memorial Committee. Dr Basu's noble mission was interrupted in 1986 with his demise.

In the 1970s, several research findings in scientific literature — particularly those concerning pain relief, like the gate control theory, endorphin-enkephalin theory of acupuncture analgesia — renewed the interest of the scientific and medical community in acupuncture. In due course, besides socially motivated acupuncture health workers, various medical graduates became interested in acupuncture and started to practise it as a system of therapy or as an adjunct to other therapeutic modalities.

It is also interesting to note that most scientific and medical institutions and agencies of India have shown an intense scientific interest towards the development and standardized application of acupuncture. The premier medical research body — the Indian Council of Medical Research (ICMR) has already identified fundamental and applied research on acupuncture as an important area of medical research. ICMR experts are giving more stress to its mechanism of action, immunomodulatory properties, and philosophical dimensions. Many other eminent medical professionals are also showing growing interest in this traditional but potentially very effective art of healing.

2

The Philosophy of Acupuncture

It is rather difficult to understand acupuncture without trying to understand Chinese medicine, and Chinese medicine can only be properly understood in the context of Chinese philosophy.

According to the Chinese view of the world, mankind is seen as living between Heaven and Earth. The energies and influences of Heaven and Earth intermingle within human beings in a dynamic balance. The air we breathe — coming from Heaven — and the food we eat — coming from Earth, combine in us to provide the energy necessary for life.

The human body is seen as the dynamic centre for this interchange. But Heaven and Earth to the Chinese are more than just producers of air and food. They represent two poles — creative and receptive. This meeting of Heaven and Earth within a person must be kept in harmony and balance. Each internal organ has

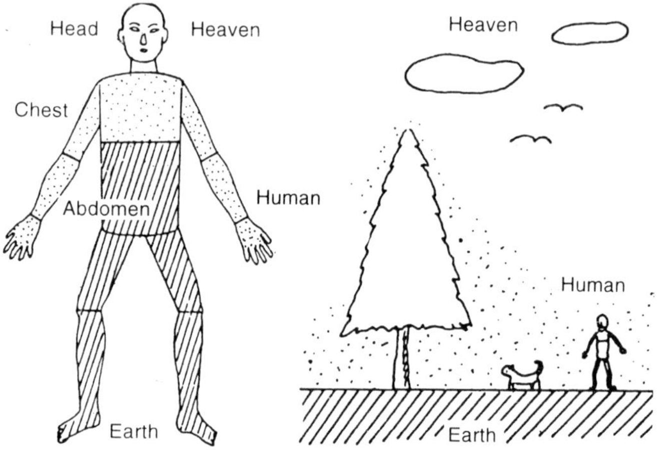

Fig. 1. Energies from Heaven and Earth Provide Human Energy

a particular function in this process, and must be able to work well and in harmony with the other organs. It is a finely-tuned system, and breakdown in any one area affects the whole human body.

Chinese philosophy lays emphasis on having a balance in all activities: between times of activity and times of rest; between expenditure of energy and nourishment; between times of excitement and times of quiet reflection. In Chinese terminology, this means balancing the *Yin* and *Yang* aspects of life.

Yin and *Yang*

Everything in the Chinese view of the world and life is related to a dynamic balance of *Yin/Yang*. They are an inseparable couple. *Yin* is the passive female principle and *Yang* is the active male counterpart. Life takes place in the alternating rhythm of *Yin/Yang*: *Yin* (night), a time of darkness and rest, gives way to *Yang* (day), a time of light and activity. Flowers open and close, the moon waxes and wanes, we wake and sleep, breathe in and breathe out. *Yin* and *Yang* together, are a constant, continuous flow of life. Their proper and balanced relationship is health; a disturbance or imbalance in this relationship is disease.

In Traditional Chinese Medicine it is this dualistic principle of perfect harmony between *Yin* and *Yang* that is the fundamental and necessary part of creation, of being, and of ideal health.

In medicine, *Yin/Yang* is used to describe and distinguish patterns of disharmony. In distinguishing illness patterns, weakness suggests *Yin*, and strength, *Yang*. The important point is that nothing is ever entirely *Yin* or *Yang*: everything contains the possibility of interchanging with its opposite. This intermingling, changing pattern of *Yin/Yang* is beautifully illustrated by the symbol of *Tai Ji* — The Great Polarity (Fig. 2). All things have a *Yin* and *Yang* aspect represented in *Tai Ji* by the light (*Yang*) and dark (*Yin*) areas. They are in balance, but this balance is fluid and changing.

The small black circle within the light area, and the small white circle within the black, demonstrate that

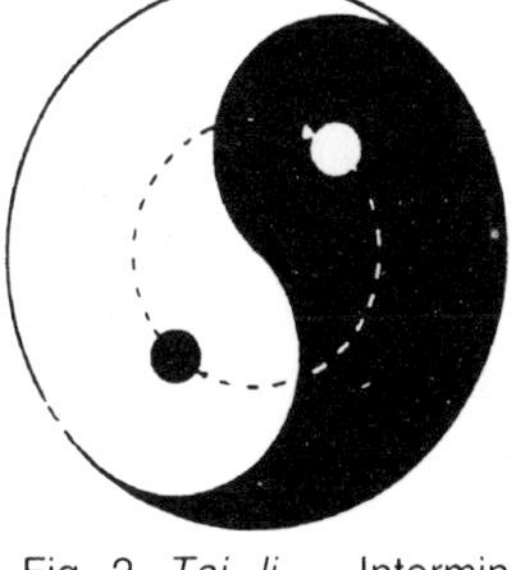

Fig. 2. *Tai Ji* — Intermingling of *Yin* and *Yang*

Yang has its root in *Yin*.
Yin has its root in *Yang*.
Without *Yin, Yang* cannot arise.
Without *Yang, Yin* cannot be born.
Yin alone cannot arise; *Yang* alone cannot grow.
Yin and *Yang* are divisible but inseparable.

— *Nei Jing*

nothing is pure *Yin* or pure *Yang*. This explains the endless variety of all life, the uniqueness of each individual. This understanding is crucial for acupuncture diagnosis and treatment. This is the principle of mutual support which can be seen in any relationship. Mutual support is complemented by mutual control. There is a counterbalancing of *Yin* with *Yang* and vice versa — a natural tendency to bring things back to normal.

Qi: Life-Giving Energy

According to Chinese philosophy, everything in the universe comprises energy. Man is an energetic being. All matter is energy. This energy in the Chinese language is called *Qi* (pronounced chee). If life is movement, *Qi* is what makes things move and is the movement itself. It is activating, enlivening, and animating. Without this movement, vibration, activity, circulation, and flow, there is no life. Chinese philosophy maintains that there is no split between energy and matter. Living things are not seen as matter activated by energy, but as energy organised into matter.

The primary function of *Qi* can be seen in all movements, whether involuntary — such as heartbeats and respiration, or voluntary — such as eating, speaking, walking, and even thinking. Life is movement and *Qi* governs it. Much of acupuncture is concerned with restoring free movement and the proper direction of such movement.

Qi flows along the energy channels just as blood flows along the blood vessels, producing warmth and supplying energy which keeps human beings alive. Although nourishment is more a function of blood, *Qi* also nourishes and maintains the organs and tissues.

Associated with this function is the role of *Qi* in increasing resistance to disease and strengthening the body's immunity.

Qi is of different types and is seen as flowing in an invisible network of channels (called meridians) and interconnections that integrate the entire energetic functioning of the body. The principal functions of *Qi* are to activate and move, to nourish, to protect, and to warm.

Where *Qi* Comes From. The Chinese say that *Qi* comes from three sources:

➤ Prenatal *Qi*. This is the *Qi* that we are born with, that we receive from our parents at conception. Different individuals may have more or less of it, which at least partly explains why some people naturally have more vitality than others, even at the earliest age. This *Qi* resides in the lower abdomen.

➤ Food *Qi*. This *Qi* is developed through the digestion of food. Healthy or poor digestion can have an immediate impact on this *Qi* and on our overall energy level.

➤ Air *Qi*. The air we breathe is the source of this *Qi*. Deep, full breathing and at least light aerobic exercise are necessary in order to have a healthy amount of air *Qi*.

The different forms of *Qi* combine in the body. If the *Qi* of an organ is weakened, the function of that organ becomes faulty or incomplete, and if *Qi* is present in excess, the result is over-functioning of the organ.

According to Traditional Chinese Medicine most illnesses are rooted in the flow of *Qi*: that is, there is either an excess or a deficiency of the vital energy in the organs and channels and either can cause illness.

The Biological Clock

The Chinese postulate that during a 24-hour cycle, the duration of peak (maximum) flow of *Qi* or the vital energy in any meridian is for a maximum of two hour period. This is illustrated in Fig. 3.

Each organ is prone to suffering from problems at the time when the maximum *Qi* is flowing through it. For example, the maximum flow of energy through the large intestine is between 5 a.m. and 7 a.m., which is why most of us pass stools early in the morning. The *Qi* flow through the lung meridian is maximum between 3-5 a.m. So often, asthma patients suffer from attacks at this hour.

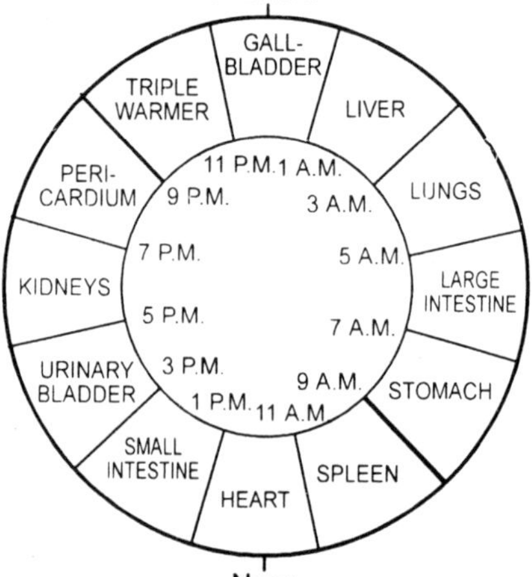

Fig. 3. The Biological Clock

This concept of a biological clock has been confirmed by research carried out during the last 30 years, which reiterates the functioning of all living beings with an internal clock.

The Meridian System

Along with the concept of *Qi*, acupuncture postulates that *Qi* or energy flows and circulates through the body in a network of meridians or channels.

There are a total of 20 meridians: 12 main, 1 front midline, 1 back midline, and 6 extra collateral meridians, through which energy flows in the body. Each of these have a body organ or system associated to it.

Meridians	*Associated Organ(s)*
1. Lung Meridian	Lungs
2. Large Intestine Meridian	Large Intestine
3. Stomach Meridian	Stomach
4. Spleen Meridian	Spleen
5. Heart Meridian	Heart
6. Small Intestine Meridian	Small Intestine
7. Urinary Bladder Meridian	Urinary Bladder
8. Kidney Meridian	Kidneys
9. Pericardium Meridian	Pericardium*
10. Triple Warmer Meridian	Triple Warmer**
11. Gall-bladder Meridian	Gall-bladder
12. Liver Meridian	Liver
13. Front Midline Meridian 14. Back Midline Meridian	These meridians are associated with the organs that lie in the centre of the body (both on the front and the back).

* The membranous sac enclosing the heart.

** The triple warmer, according to acupuncture principles/texts, consists of the 3 body cavities: chest cavity — heart and lungs; abdominal cavity — all organs of the digestive system; the pelvic cavity — the genitalia and urinary organs.

The front midline meridian (*Yin*) and the back midline meridian (*Yang*) control the energy flow in all the meridians and correlate their activities.

The 14 meridians (12 main and 2 midline) do not merge, though they do cross, one on top of the other. Each meridian is a totally separate entity.

The six remaining extra meridians are not associated with any specific organ but connect portions of the main meridians, which come into play for complicated health conditions.

This interlacing network of meridians is the crux of traditional acupuncture. The Chinese themselves have compared the flow of *Qi* through the meridian system to water irrigating the land: feeding, nourishing, and sustaining the substances through which it flows. It is similar in some ways to the blood circulation and nervous system. It is invisible to the eye, but the flow of *Qi* through the meridians can be sensed from its effects by a trained practitioner and has been charted for more than 2,000 years.

The meridian lines are divided into negative and positive forces — or *Yin* and *Yang*.

The *Yin* Meridians. The front side of the body is the *Yin* side. If you stand with your feet turned out and your arms raised above your head, as shown in Fig. 4a, the flow of the *Yin* meridians becomes clear. There are six *Yin* meridians, three in the legs and three in the arms. The three *Yin* meridians which start from the toes ascend towards the centre of the body while the other three meridians which start from the centre of the body move upwards towards the fingertips.

The *Yang* Meridians. The back side of the body is the *Yang* side. If you stand with your feet turned out and your arms raised above your head, as shown in Fig. 4b, the flow of the *Yang* meridians becomes clear. There are six *Yang* meridians, three in the legs and three in the arms. The three *Yang* meridians which start at the top of the head and face descend towards the earth while the other three meridians which start at the top of the fingertips descend towards the centre of the body.

It is important to know if a meridian is *Yin* or *Yang* to find the direction in which the energy is flowing. An acupuncturist works with the energy flow or against it, depending on whether he wants to increase or decrease the energy level of a patient.

'A skilful doctor cures illness when there is no sign of disease and thus the disease never comes.'

Huai Nan Zi, 120 BC

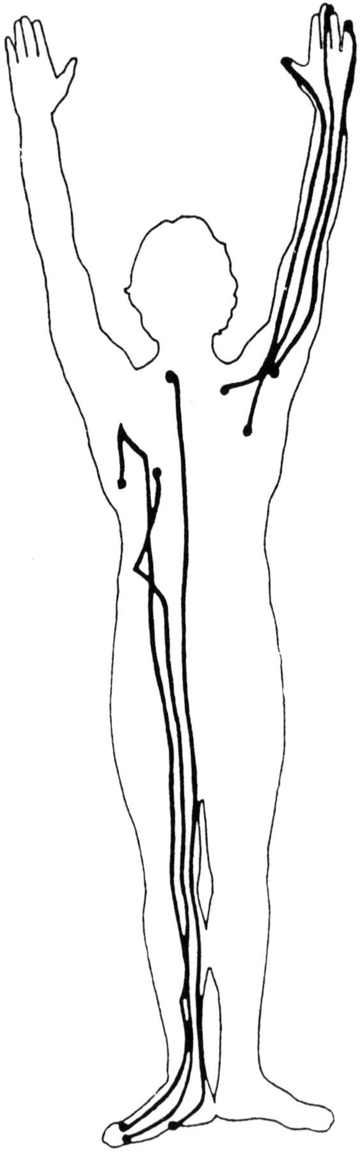

Fig. 4A. The Six *Yin* Meridians

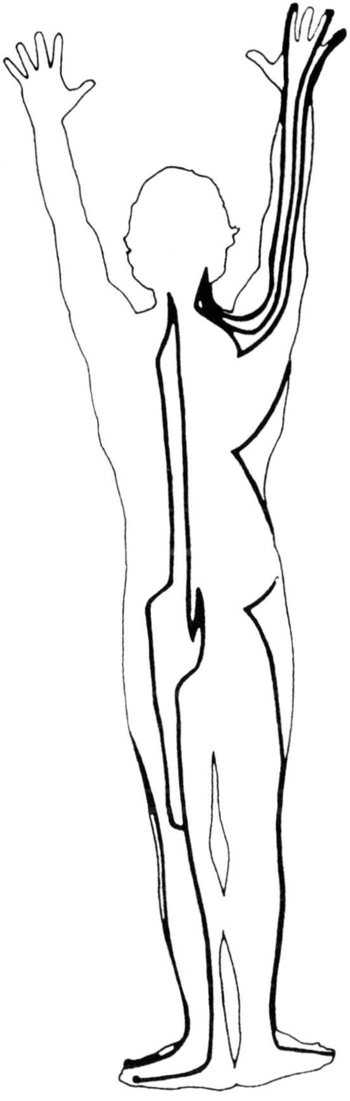

Fig. 4B. The Six *Yang* Meridians

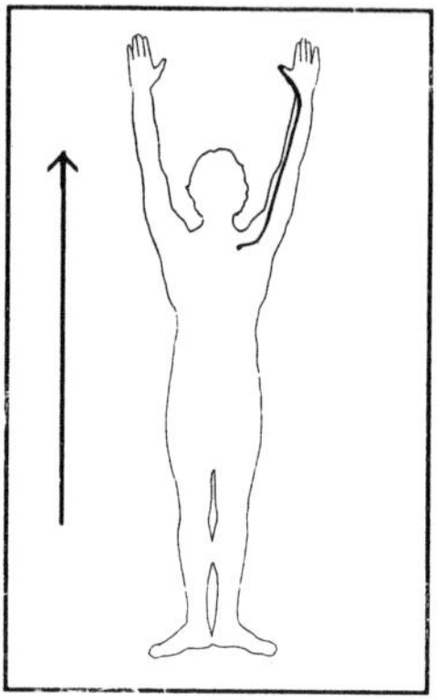

Hand *Taiyin* is a *Yin* Meridian

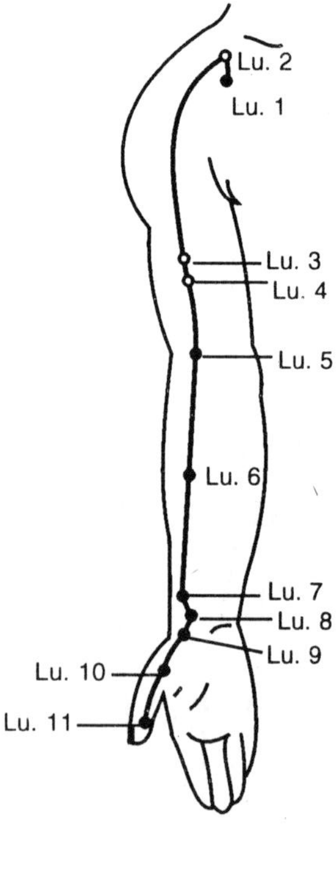

Acupuncture Points on Hand *Taiyin* — the Lung Meridian (Lu)
• Frequently Used Points 8 o Ordinary Points 3

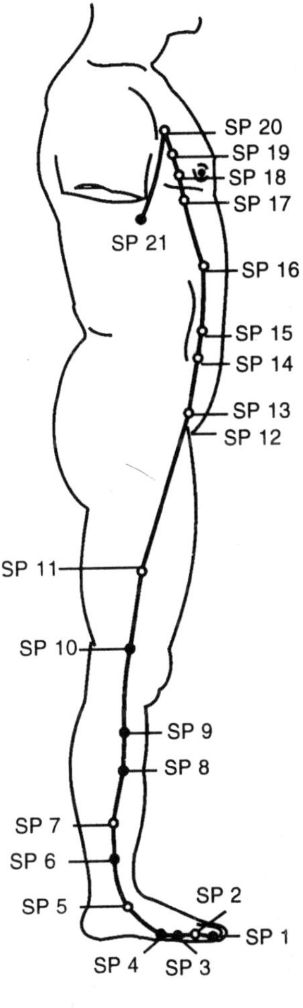

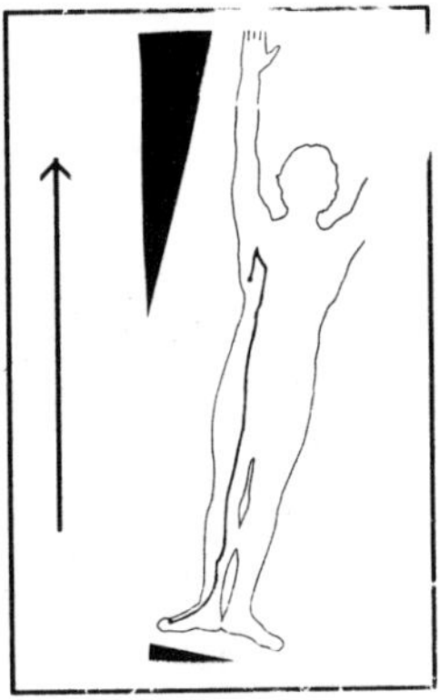

Foot *Taiyin* is a *Yin* Meridian

Acupuncture Points on Foot *Taiyin* — the Spleen Meridian (SP)

• Frequently Used Points 8 ○ Ordinary Points 13

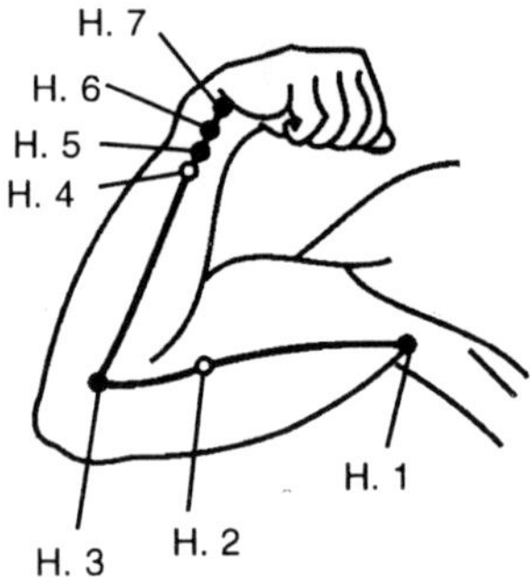

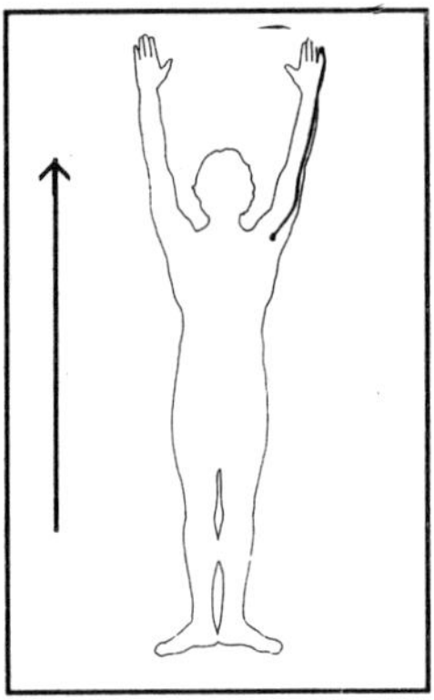

Hand *Shaoyin* is a *Yin* Meridian

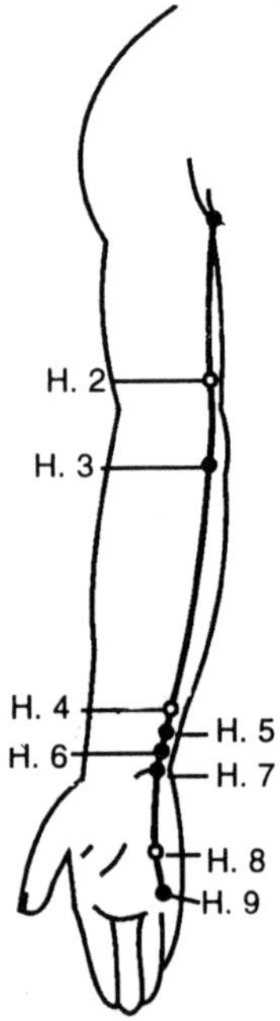

Acupuncture Points on Hand *Shaoyin* — the Heart Meridian (H)
• Frequently Used Points 6 o Ordinary Points 3

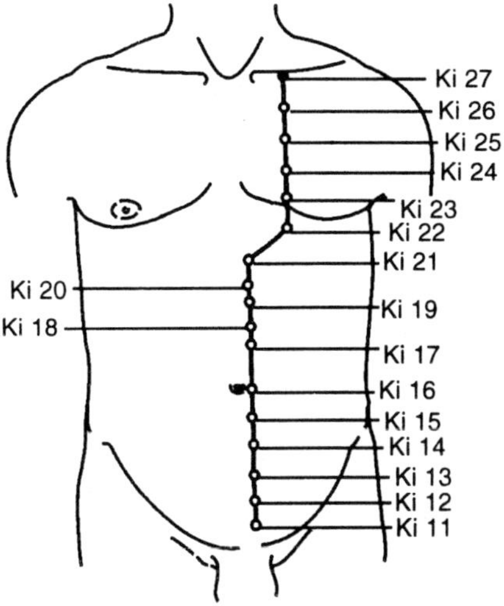

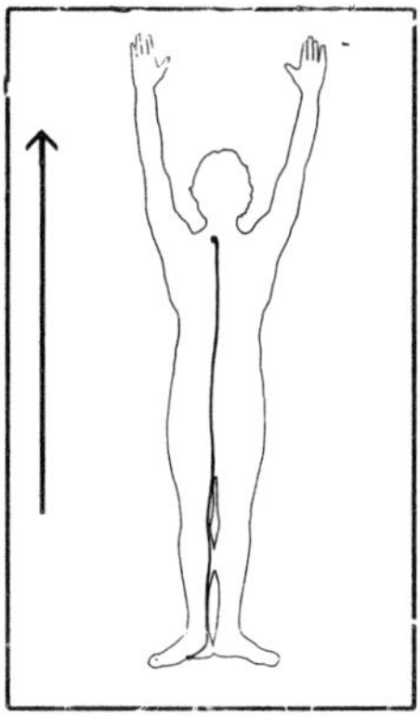

Foot *Shaoyin* is a *Yin* Meridian.

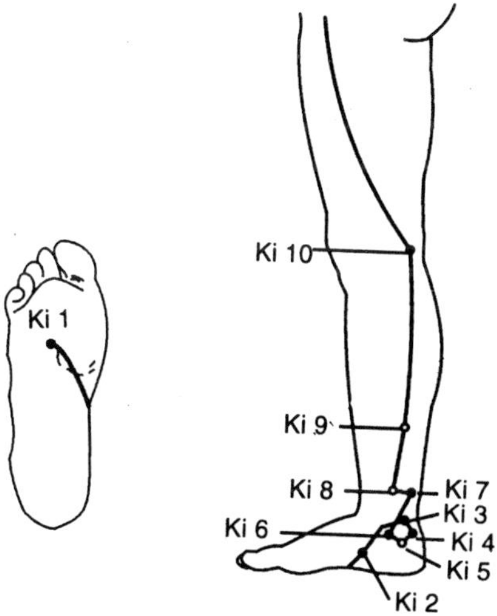

Acupuncture Points on Foot *Shaoyin* — the Kidney Meridian (Ki)
• Frequently Used Points 8 o Ordinary Points 19

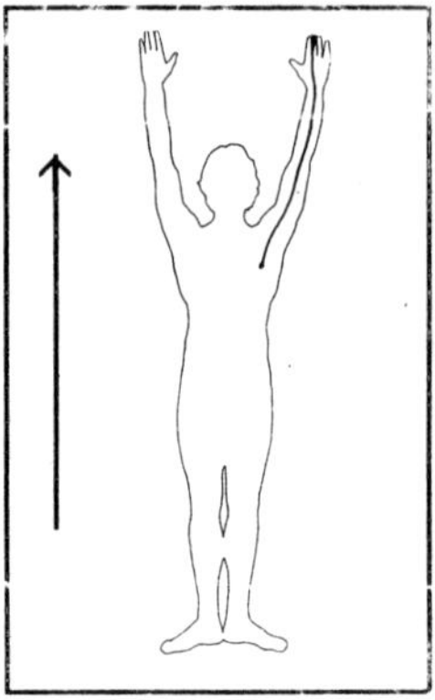

Hand *Jueyin* is a *Yin* Meridian

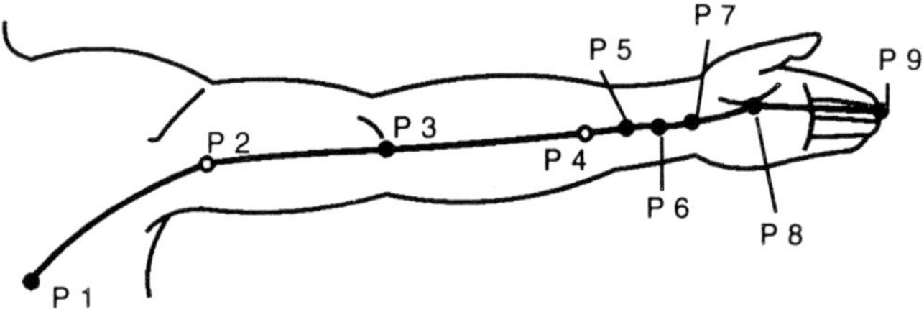

Acupuncture Points on *Hand Jueyin* — the Pericardium Meridian (P)
• Frequently Used Points 7 o Ordinary Points 2

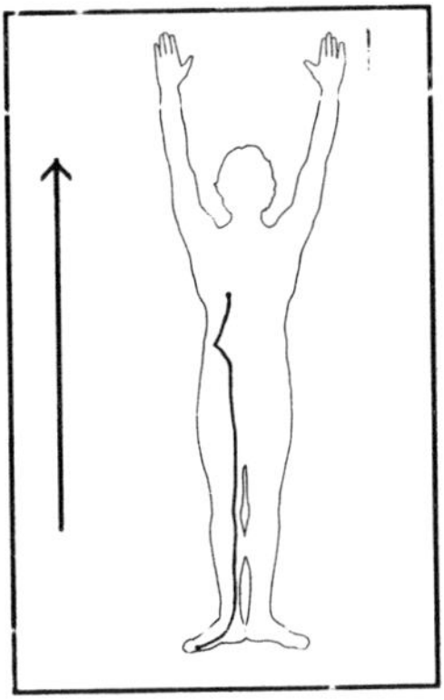

Foot *Jueyin* is a *Yin* Meridian

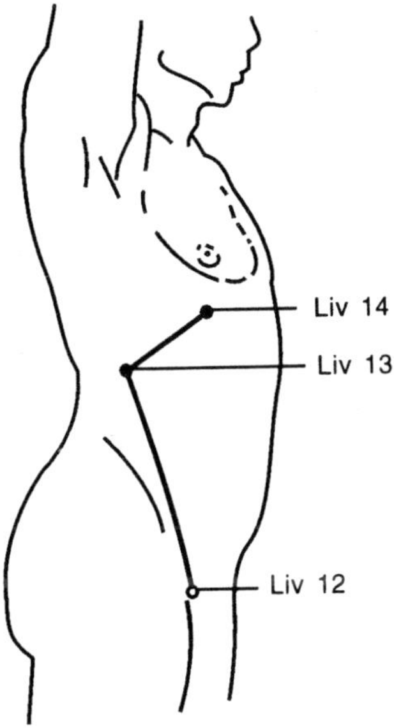

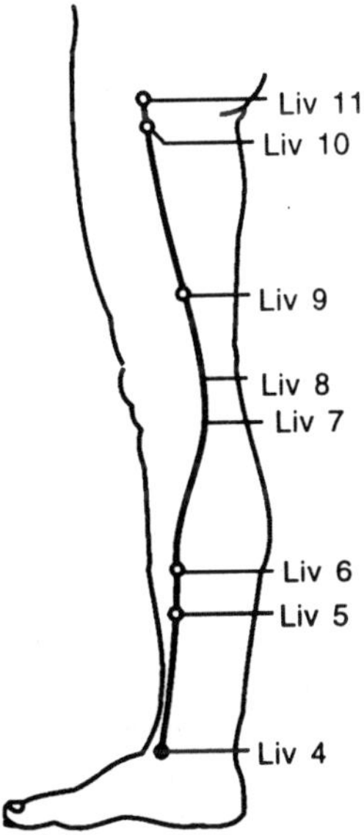

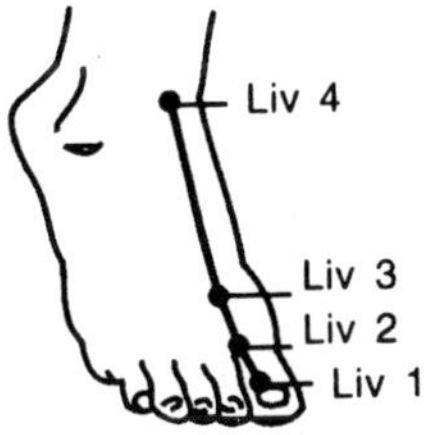

Acupuncture Points on Foot *Jueyin* — the Liver Meridian (Liv)
• Frequently Used Points 5 o Ordinary Points 6

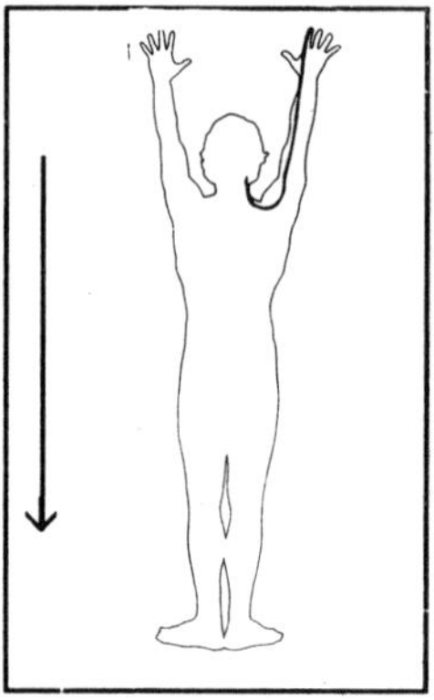

Hand *Yangming* is a *Yang* Meridian

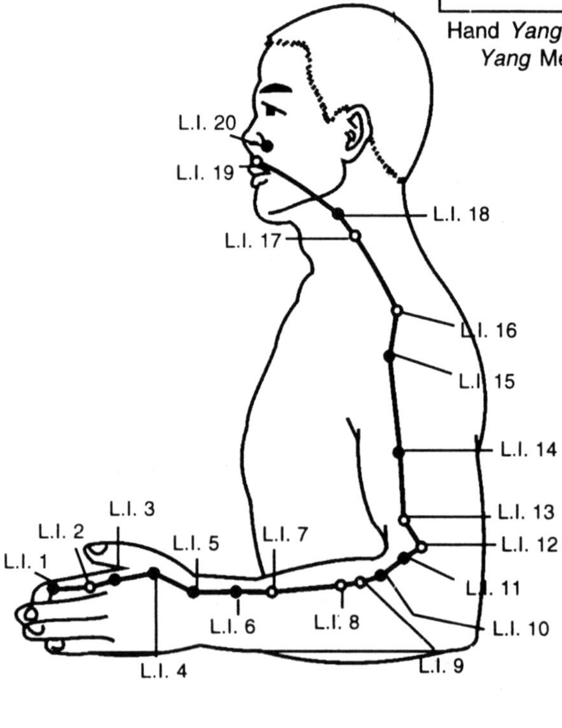

Acupuncture Points on Hand *Yangming* — Large Intestine Meridian (Li)

• Frequently Used Points 11 o Ordinary Points 9

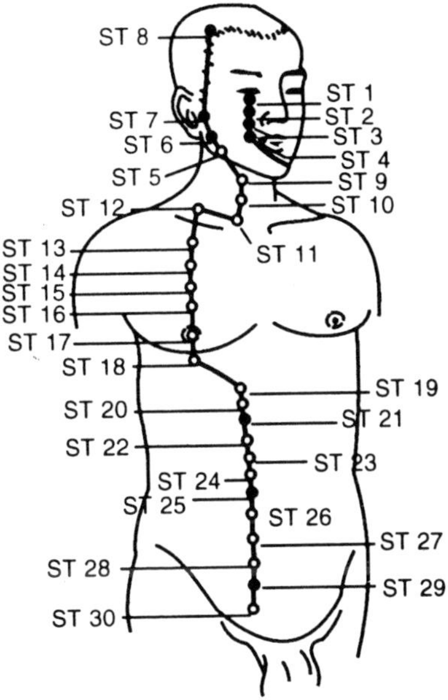

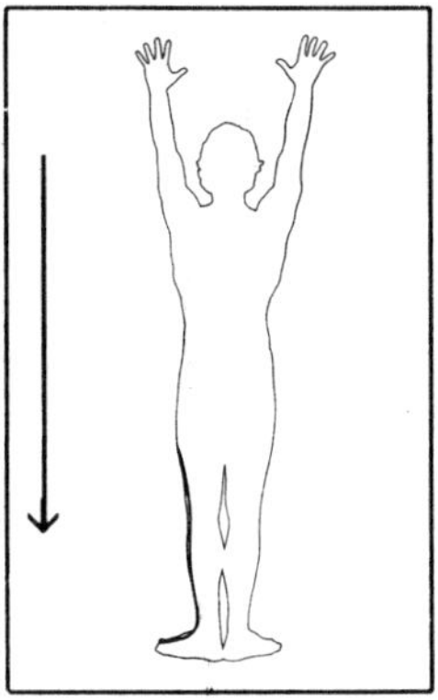

Foot *Yangming* is a *Yang* Meridian

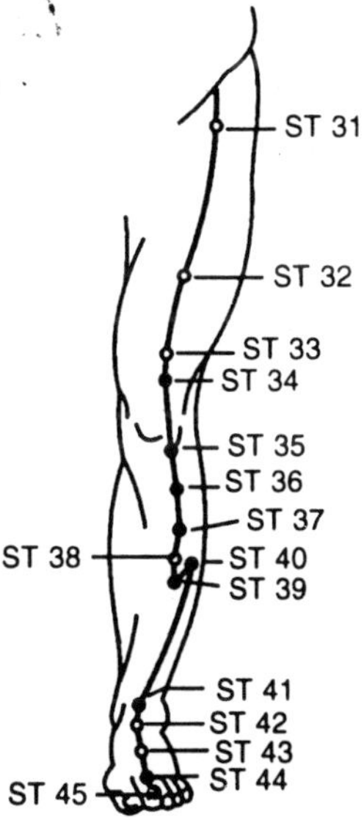

Acupuncture Points on Foot *Yangming* — the Stomach Meridian (ST)

• Frequently Used Points 18 o Ordinary Points 27

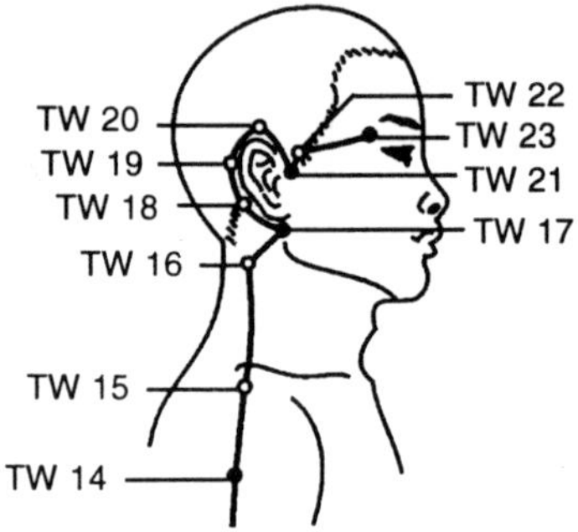

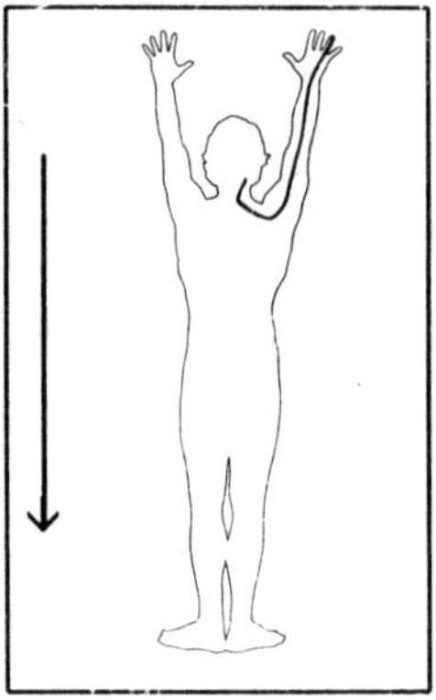

Hand *Shaoyang* is a *Yang* Meridian

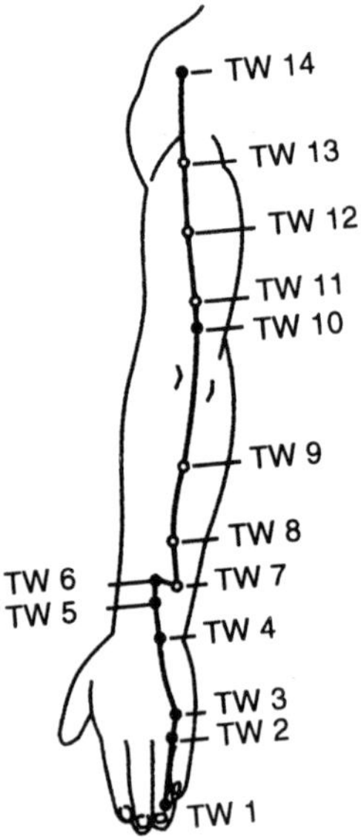

Acupuncture Points on Hand *Shaoyang* — Triple Warmer Meridian (TW)

• Frequently Used Points 11   o Ordinary Points 12

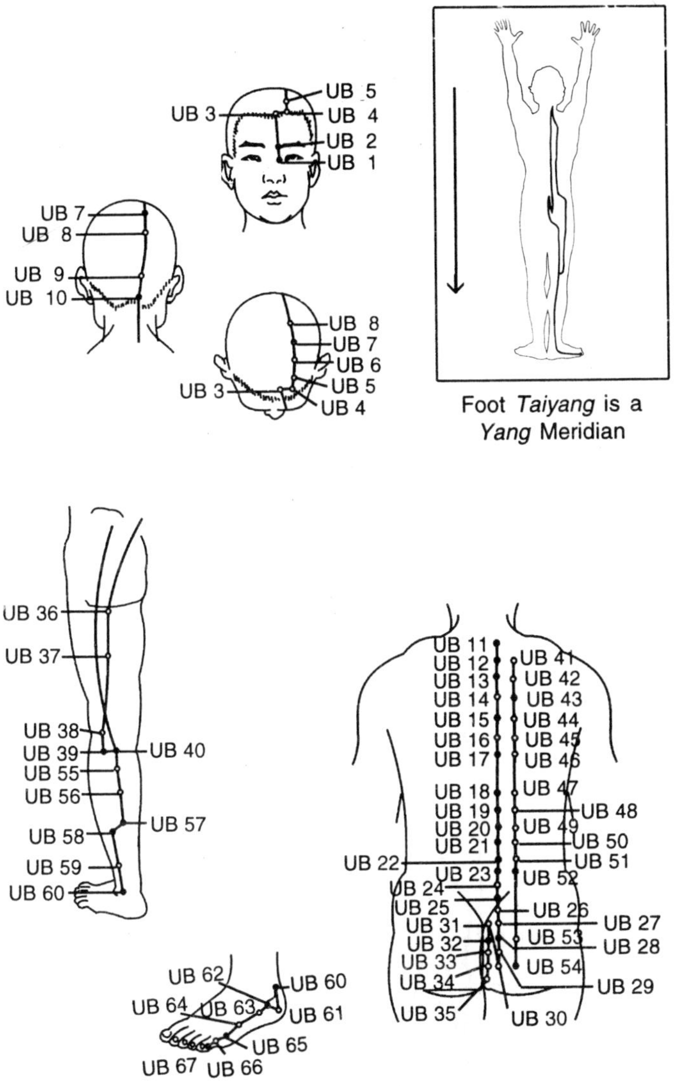

Foot *Taiyang* is a *Yang* Meridian

Acupuncture Points on Foot *Taiyang* — Urinary Bladder Meridian (UB)
● Frequently Used Points 29 o Ordinary Points 38

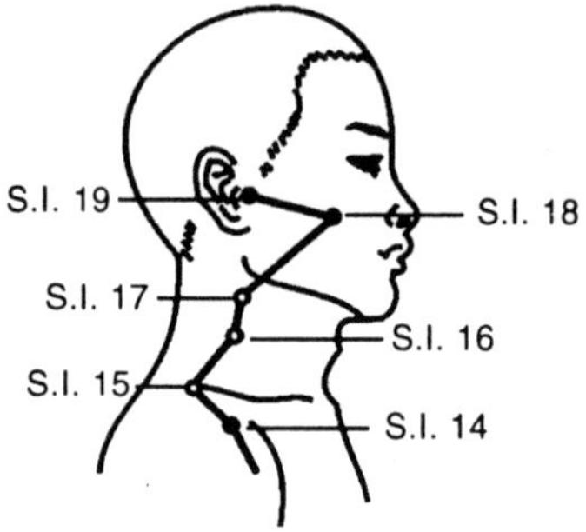

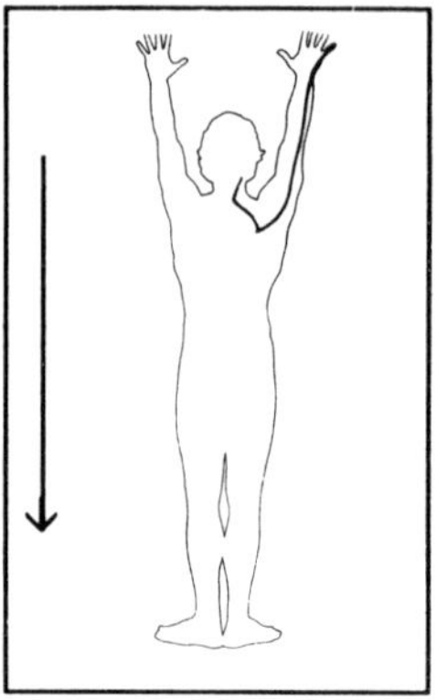

Hand *Taiyang* is a *Yang* Meridian.

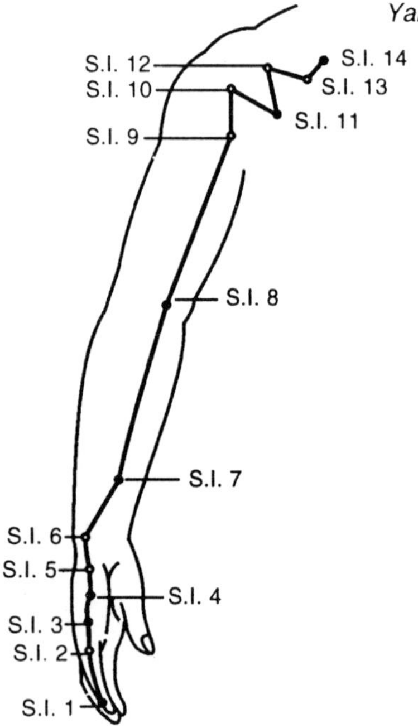

Acupuncture Points on Hand *Taiyang* — Small Intestine Meridian (SI)
• Frequently Used Points 9 o Ordinary Points 10

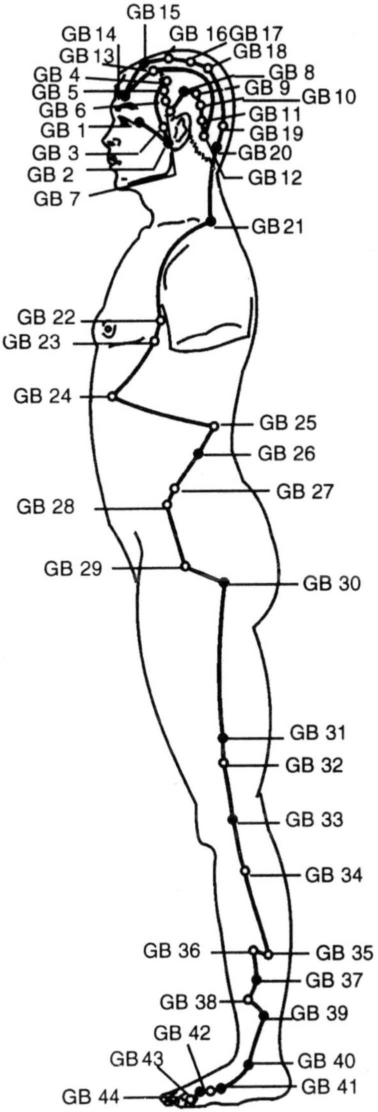

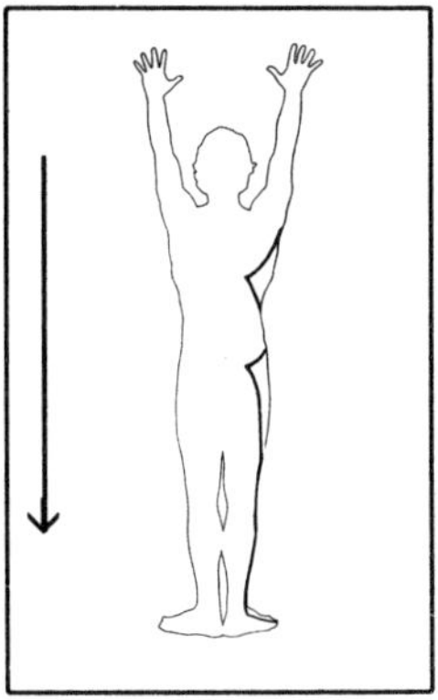

Foot *Shaoyang* is a *Yang* Meridian

Acupuncture Points on Foot *Shaoyang* — Gall-Bladder Meridian (GB)

• Frequently Used Points 18 o Ordinary Points 26

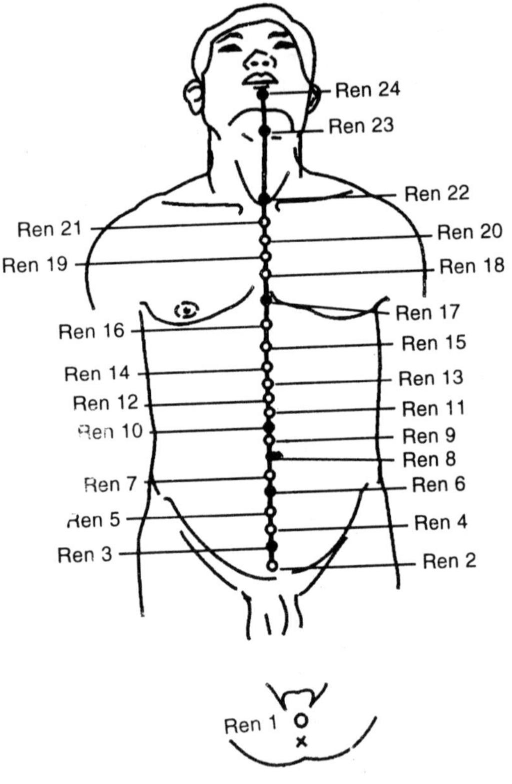

Acupuncture Points on *Ren* Meridian — Front Midline Meridian (*Ren*)
• Frequently Used Points 8 o Ordinary Points 16

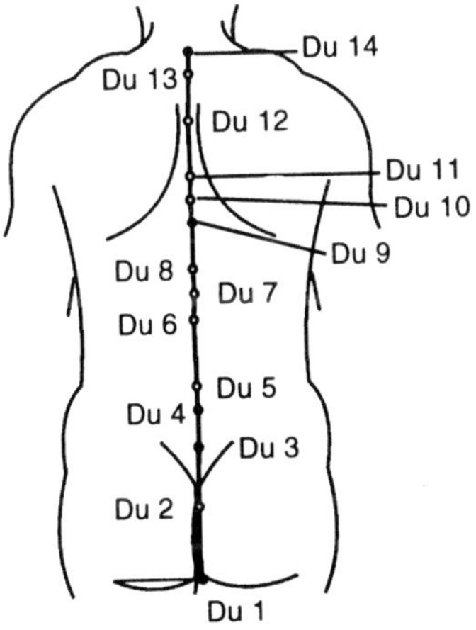

Acupuncture Points on *Du* Meridian — Back Midline Meridian (*Du*)
• Frequently Used Points 12 o Ordinary Points 16

The Flow of *Qi*. The 12 main meridians are coupled into 6 pairs. Each pair consists of 1 *Yin* meridian and 1 *Yang* meridian which are interconnected through a vessel known as a luoconnecting vessel.

Coupling of Main Meridians	*Flow of Qi*
1. Hand *Taiyin*	Lungs
(Lung Meridian)	↓
Hand *Yangming*	Large Intestine
(Large Intestine Meridian)	↓
2. Foot *Yangming*	Stomach
(Stomach Meridian)	↓
Foot *Taiyin*	Spleen
(Spleen Meridian)	↓
3. Hand *Shaoyin*	Heart
(Heart Meridian)	↓
Hand *Taiyang*	Small Intestine
(Small Intestine Meridian)	↓
4. Foot *Taiyang*	Urinary Bladder
(Urinary Bladder Meridian)	↓
Foot *Shaoyin*	Kidneys
(Kidney Meridian)	↓
5. Hand *Jueyin*	Pericardium
(Pericardium Meridian)	↓
Hand *Shaoyang*	Triple Warmer
(Triple Warmer Meridian)	↓
6. Foot *Shaoyang*	Gall-bladder
(Gall-bladder Meridian)	↓
Foot *Jueyin*	Liver
(Liver Meridian)	

The flow of energy starts from the lungs and goes through the large intestine, stomach, spleen, heart, small intestine, urinary bladder, kidneys, pericardium, triple warmer, gall-bladder, and liver, in that order, and then goes back to the lungs to start the cycle again. In this manner the network of meridians links the internal organs, body surface, the head, and the limbs into one integrated whole. This integration gives acupuncture the tremendous flexibility of being able to treat illness in any part of the body from another part of the body. For example, an acupuncturist can treat a problem like backache from points on the hand, ear, face, scalp, foot, or back.

Despite the fact that meridians possess names of their related organs, the excess or deficiency of *Qi* in a meridian does not always indicate the existence of a disease in that particular organ.

Acupuncture Points

There are over 2,000 acupuncture points recognized by the practitioners, and of these about 365 points, which are commonly used, are on the 14 main meridians. Each meridian has a series of 'command' points, which are located between the elbows and fingertips, and the knees and toes. The command points at the tips of the fingers and toes are called 'Well' or 'Spring' points, whereas the points located at the knees and elbows are called 'Sea' points. These acupuncture points are the most frequently used in treatment as their energetic qualities are very specific and the flow of *Qi* in the meridians is most dynamic at the four extremities.

In addition to the 'command' points, specific acupuncture points on the trunk relate to a particular organ function, and also tend to be frequently used. Some acupuncture points are the meeting of meridian pathways, others the junction with an internal pathway of the meridian: some tend to move energy towards the interior of the body, others bring energy to the surface. All acupuncture points have a specific anatomical location including on the ears, nose, hands, feet, and the scalp. These acupuncture points are reached and stimulated by inserting fine needles through the body's skin. When any specific point or points are 'needled', the *Qi* flowing through the meridian on which the acupuncture point lies is affected. The *Qi* or the energy flowing through that meridian is either increased or reduced or even blocked, depending on the treatment required. Treatment at these points can prevent development of or treat a disease in the related organs. Each acupuncture point can be used to treat several diseases as it influences several organs, both through the main meridians and their collaterals.

The Holistic Approach

It is important to recognize that acupuncture is only one part of the whole spectrum of Traditional Chinese Medicine. This also includes treatment with herbs, corrections in diet, massage, and exercise. These methods of treatment may be used in conjunction with acupuncture or even instead of it. Acupuncture is not, therefore, a system of medicine in isolation. It should be seen as one major method of treatment within a complete system that has a different perspective on health from that of orthodox Western medicine.

Not surprisingly, being an integrated approach, it is much more demanding to practice. No symptom is dealt with in relative isolation, but is constantly related to the whole until a complete picture of physical, mental, and emotional harmony is established.

3

Diagnosis in Acupuncture

One of the fundamental tenets of the Chinese philosophy of life is the belief that the energy present in the universe alternates between *Yin* and *Yang*. A later refinement of the *Yin/Yang* concept was introduced around 400 BC — that of *Wu Xing* or the five elements. It was believed that when creation took place, the *Yin* and *Yang* brought forth the five elements of water, wood, fire, earth, and metal which represent the five aspects of energy. According to the Chinese, these five elements are present in the human body and good physical, mental, and spiritual health is dependent on a state of equilibrium between these elements. The interaction of *Yin* and *Yang* ensures that the proportion of these elements is correctly maintained in the body.

The meaning and significance of these elements in acupuncture diagnosis and treatment is discussed in this chapter.

Qi and the Five Elements (*Wu Xing*) in the Human Body

According to the Chinese, each of the five elements — water, wood, fire, earth, and metal — has a psychological link with a specific emotion and a physiological link with a particular organ of the body. They firmly believe that good health is dependent upon harmonious equilibrium between the five elements, the emotions, and the physical body. An imbalance in any of the elements and/or emotions affects the normal working of the human body and the state of good health.

According to them the correct balance of assertiveness, joy, calmness, sympathy, and respect is essential. Excessive emotions such as anger, joy, excitement, obsession, prolonged grief, fearfulness or anxiety, or similar enhanced emotional states are the internal factors which lead to poor health or even disease. More precisely, they are manifestations of imbalances in the five elements caused by internal emotional factors, and therefore, health can be improved, or disease cured by addressing the elements in the body.

It is against this fundamental belief in the inter-relationship and interdependence between the elements, the human emotions, and the state of health, that there is a need to understand the role and importance of the five elements.

Water is basic to life on this planet. In man the fluids of the body nourish and maintain the health of every cell and if these fluids become toxic, the result is disease. The fluids are manifested as blood, lymph, mucus, semen, and fats. Any imbalance in the flow of liquids (caused by excessive fear) leads to deficiencies in the functioning of the kidneys and the urinary bladder.

Elements and their Psychological and Physiological Associations

Elements	*Emotions*	*Organs*
Water	Fear	Urinary bladder, Kidneys
Wood	Anger	Gall-bladder, Liver
Fire	Joy	Heart, Small intestine
Earth	Stability/ Mental well-being	Stomach, Spleen
Metal	Grief/ Melancholy	Lungs, Large intestine

The latter are responsible for healthy teeth and hair, good hearing, and sexual vitality.

Wood is the element or energy responsible for digestion, heartbeats, respiration, and basic metabolism. These functions carry on in a healthy manner unless the individual is filled with excessive anger or suppresses it totally. In such a condition, there is an imbalance in the *wood*, which results in a malfunctioning of the liver and the gall-bladder. Consequently these organs fail to provide the required supply of energy to the muscles, tendons and ligaments, and to keep the eyes healthy.

Fire, as the name suggests, influences the working of the circulatory system and the power of speech. Excessive pleasure or joy or a lack of them affect the psyche of a man. When the emotions are in balance, the flow of energy is well-regulated and there is a healthy circulation. If there is an imbalance in *fire*, there will be a malfunctioning of the heart and small intestine — its related organs, thus disturbing the circulation.

Earth makes an individual mentally stable and contented. He experiences physical and social well-being. The other four elements of water, wood, fire, and metal are all responsible for the balance of *earth*; when all the emotions are in balance, only then is a state of stability achieved. When the *earth* is imbalanced, there is a malfunctioning of its related organs — the spleen and the stomach. The connective tissues in the body become undernourished and the sense of taste is adversely affected.

Metal is that form of energy which is responsible for the working of the lungs and the large intestine — that is, healthy respiration and assimilation of food. However, excessive or suppressed grief or melancholy upsets the flow in this energy, resulting in malfunctioning of the lungs and large intestine. The nose and sense of smell. the condition of the skin, the assimilation and elimination of food and other substances are adversely affected.

The *Sheng* and *Ke* Cycles

Just a everything is *Yin/Yang*, or can be expressed in terms of *Yin/Yang*, so also, in a broader sense, everything in Chinese medicine can be expressed in terms of the five elements. In the same sense, all health issues are seen in terms of interrelationships between these five elements — Is the Earth weak? Is the Wood too strong? By themselves none of these statements are important unless we study the interrelationships between these elements. It is the interrelationship and balance that is important so that the five elements integrate and move in harmony and balance. Their interaction is governed by definite relationships known as *Sheng* and *Ke* cycles.

Sheng means to create or produce. Hence each element gives birth to the one succeeding it. So Water produces

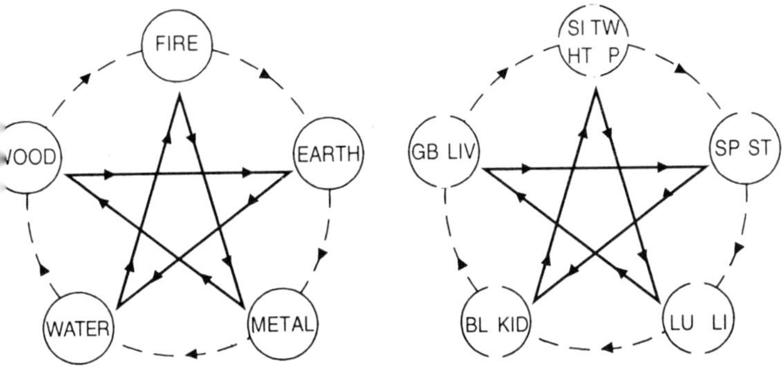

Fig. 5. Relationship between Elements and Organs in the *Sheng* and *Ke* Cycles
Cycle of Creation ——▶—— = *Sheng*
Cycle of Control — ▶ — = *Ke*

Key HT-heart, SI-small intestine, P-pericardium, TW-triple warmer, SP-spleen, ST-stomach, LU-lungs, LI-large intestine, KID-kidneys, BL-urinary bladder, LIV-liver, GB-gall-bladder

Wood: Wood produces Fire; Fire produces Earth; Earth produces Metal; and Metal produces Water. A problem in any organ of the body is attributed to it not being properly nourished by its creator or promoter. A lung disorder, for example, is seen as a failure of the spleen to transmit vital energy or *Qi* to the lungs. This explanation is consistent with Western medical thinking.

Ke means control. In the *Ke* cycle, each element controls *not* the next, but one following the next element. So Water controls Fire; Wood controls Earth; Fire controls Metal; Earth controls Water; and Metal controls Wood.

In order to have harmony and good health, both the cycles must operate: overproduction of *Qi* in any channel leads to an excess of *Qi* there, whereas insufficient production results in stagnation. Therefore production (*Sheng*) and control (*Ke*) must go hand in hand. When the balance breaks down, the result is illness.

Diagnostic Criteria in Chinese Medicine

The diagnostic system of Chinese medicine developed on the basis of the philosophical system of *Yin/Yang* and the five-element theory. There are eight diagnostic criteria grouped into four categories, according to which a disease is classified. These are:

1. Interior or Exterior
2. Deficiency or Excess
3. Cold or Heat
4. *Yin* or *Yang*

Interior or Exterior. Internal illnesses are disharmonious states of the internal organs. They are frequently chronic in nature, being characterized by pain in the thorax or abdomen, raised body temperature, and disturbances of gastro-intestinal functions such as diarrhoea and nausea. Internal illnesses are often caused by extreme feelings such as anxiety, fear, sadness or excitement, or by inadequate or contaminated food.

External illnesses are characterized by disturbances of the channels and their branches, especially in the peripheral regions and on the surface of the body. External illnesses are usually characterized by acute pain in the extremities, joints, or head, and by susceptibility to climatic factors. They are usually manifested as peripheral neuralgia or localised joint disease. Chinese medicine considers that these are caused by external pathogenic climatic influences like cold, heat, dampness, wind, or dryness.

Deficiency or Excess. Deficiency illnesses are characterized by deficiency of the vital energy — *Qi*. Deficiency-induced illnesses lead to hypofunction of the organ systems. Typical symptoms are excessive exhaustion, dizziness, motor retardation, low blood pressure, sudden sweating, and deficiency of body fluids. Deficiency illnesses are generally chronic. The most usual cause is exhaustion of the *Qi*, following the action of internal pathogenic influences over a long period.

Excess illnesses are characterized by excess of *Qi* or blood in the organs and channels. Typical symptoms are acute pain, cramps, hypertension, increased muscle tone, and increased secretion of body fluids. Prominent indications are redness of the face and a strong pulse.

Cold or Heat. Cold illnesses occur when external pathogenic cold takes effect in a body in which *Qi* is weak. In these circumstances, the typical cold-type symptoms manifest themselves, such as a feeling of cold, cold extremities, and pallor. Cold illnesses are usually chronic.

Heat illnesses are caused basically by the increased *Yang* activity of the *Qi* in the body. Typical heat-type symptoms include high body temperature, redness, pain, and agitation.

Yin Disorders	*Yang Disorders*
Internal illnesses	External illnesses
Deficiency illnesses	Excess illnesses
Cold illnesses	Heat illnesses
Chronic illnesses	Acute illnesses
Examples	
Hypothermia	Fever
Hypotension	Hypertension
Depression	Excitement, mania
Pain, chronic	Pain, acute
Exhaustion	Hyperactivity
Feeling cold	Feeling hot
Asthma, chronic	Asthma, acute
Eczema, generalized	Eczema, localized
Joint pains, chronic	Swoolen red joints, acute

Yin or *Yang*. *Yin* or *Yang* are the categories that have universal validity and are applicable to all phenomena. Thus deficiency of *Qi*, cold illnesses, and internal illnesses are *Yin* criteria, while excess of *Qi,* heat illnesses, and external illnesses are *Yang* criteria. Also there are illnesses which are entirely *Yin* or *Yang* in nature.

Stages of Diagnosis

In acupuncture, diseases are rarely given names as they are in Western medicine. For instance two patients with an identically named disease may be treated in a different way according to their particular pattern of symptoms and energy imbalances. In fact, as soon as the patient walks through the door, the diagnosis begins.

The practitioner notes the way the patient walks and sits, observes his facial expressions and so on, before beginning to ask questions. In fact, questioning is only a part of the traditional Chinese method of acupuncture and is sometimes considered the least important. Examination for diagnosis is actually divided into four stages: looking, listening and smelling, asking, and touching.

Looking. This part of the diagnosis begins as soon as the patient enters the consultation room. It is most important to the acupuncturist to assess the *spirit* of the patient and this is seen by the way the latter walks and moves, his general bearing, facial expressions, and responses. Observation of the tongue is possibly the most developed form of the 'looking' aspect of diagnosis.

Listening and Smelling. The most important points in this aspect of diagnosis are the sound of the voice, the breathing, smells of the body and its excretions.

Asking. Questions relating to the physical and emotional aspects of the patient are important. An emotional upset or bereavement before the onset of a particular problem may provide the most important clue to understanding a particular pattern of disharmony. Similarly, a surgical operation may have affected the present complaint by interrupting the flow of energy along the meridian pathways.

Other important questions to be asked concern sensations of heat and cold; perspiration and whether this occurs during the day or at night; headaches — when they occur and in what part of the head; urination and defecation, including frequency of bladder movements, and any tendency towards constipation or diarrhoea. Women are asked details about their menstrual cycles.

Touching. Palpation involves touching local areas of the body (which may be painful) to feel for heat, cold, swelling, tightness, or lack of skin tone.

Pulse Reading: Feeling the pulse is part of touching. In the category of touching, taking the pulse at the radial artery in the wrist is considered to be the most important, and is often the acupuncturist's main diagnostic tool.

The pulse is taken at both wrists and in three positions, by the index, middle, and ring finger. The index finger is placed closest to the wrist, the middle finger placed level with the bony protuberance of the radius bone on the outside of the wrist, and the ring finger placed farthest from the wrist. These three pulse positions correspond to the upper, middle, and lower areas of the body, with the position nearest to the wrist representing the upper portion of the body.

Two kinds of pulse readings are taken at these points and represent different parts of the body/organs, as explained earlier. A pulse is considered superficial if it appears to jump up from the surface of the skin and if it is felt only with strong pressure it is classified as deep. A healthy pulse is felt easily with only slight pressure. It fills all three positions on the wrist and has an even, rhythmic flow. Care must be taken to place the fingers correctly, and in proportion to the patient's body. A child's pulse, for example, is much closer together than an adult's, and that of a small-framed adult differs from the pulse of a larger, fatter adult.

It is important that the patient is relaxed before the pulse is taken. He or she is often asked to lie quietly for a few minutes to enable the pulse to be normal.

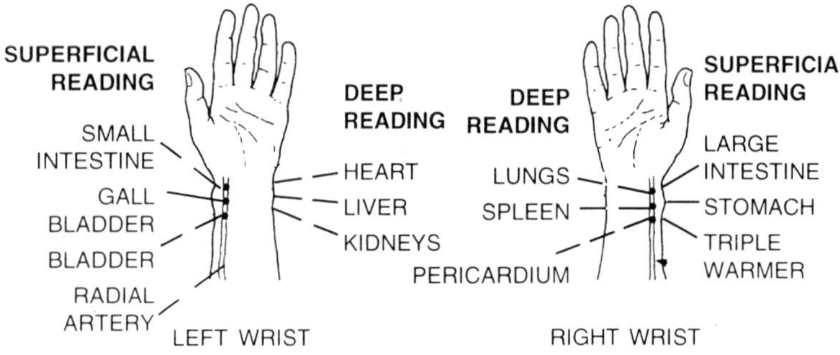

Fig. 6. Pulse Diagnosis

Traditionally, there are 28 pulse qualities, and the practitioner has to keep all of these in mind as he or she takes the pulse. The qualities are descriptions of the way the pulse feels to the fingertip, and include such categories as deep or superficial, full or empty, tight or wiry, slippery or choppy. More than any other method of diagnosis, pulse-taking requires skill and practice, and a particular sensitivity and concentration.

4

Positive Effects of Acupuncture

The underlying philosophy and objective of acupuncture is to restore a person's health, balance, and harmony on all levels — physical, mental, emotional, and spiritual — by stimulating the body's internal healing powers. The concept is holistic. A person is seen as a whole rather than as a biological machine afflicted by a series of different or isolated symptoms. With a holistic philosophy of health, which is person — rather than disease — oriented, gaining widespread acceptance outside China, the focus of research and study of the benefits of acupuncture has also changed. The question is no longer what disorders acupuncture can treat. Rather, the question being asked now is when is acupuncture *not* helpful.

This confidence has been further strengthened with medical scientists being able to understand the mechanism of action of acupuncture. Considerable evidence has emerged in the last 15-20 years on the scientific principles and mechanisms through which acupuncture works. This is further reflected in the major medical colleges and hospitals all over the world opening their doors and including acupuncture as an effective mode of treatment.

From the patient's point of view, it is not so important to understand why or how acupuncture works, as to know that it does work and works well. It is a safe, effective, and time-tested method of treatment, which in expert hands, yields miraculous results. More importantly, acupuncture is able to cure several chronic ailments which have no remedy in any other system of medicine. Some of the widely practiced applications of acupuncture are discussed here.

Pain Relief. One of the best known and widely acclaimed effect of acupuncture is relief from pain, that is, its analgesic effect. Acupuncture can provide relief from pain irrespective of its cause. This effect of acupuncture has been used to provide analgesia for many minor and major surgeries. Thousands of women all over the world have been spared the agony of labour pains by the use of acupuncture. This aspect of acupuncture has received great publicity in recent years.

How Acupuncture Controls Pain? The sensation of pain from any part of the body is carried to the thalamus, the area of the brain which perceives pain.

The pain impulses travel somewhat slowly till they reach a mechanism in the nervous system called 'the Gate'. When the Gate is bombarded with too many impulses, it closes and prevents the pain impulses from reaching the brain. This mechanism is known as the Gate Control Theory.

Another theory maintains that when acupuncture is performed, morphine-like substances called *endorphins* and *enkephalins* present in the body increase in number and block the ability of the brain to perceivepain.

Research conducted so far has led to the conclusion that acupuncture is able to relieve pain primarily through these two mechanisms. Further research in this field however continues.

Treatment of Neurological Disorders. Acupuncture is also known to stimulate muscle recovery, particularly in patients of paralytic strokes and facial paralysis. Pressureor irritation of the acupuncture points transmits repair messages to the brain. These are relayed to the centre which monitors body repair and mobilizes appropriate mechanisms.

Every organ has a related area of skin which lies adjacent to it. A dysfunction in any organ of the body gets manifested on the area of skin which becomes either painful or unduly sensitive. Inflammation of the stomach is reflected in the abdominal area above the navel; if the inflammation is in the small intestine, the area of pain is lower; and if in the colon, it is lower still. The acupuncture points of the affected organs have corresponding points in their adjoining skin areas, thus indicating that acupuncture depends upon these neural connections to promote healing. It is now universally agreed that acupuncture works through the nervous system. This explains the reason why acupuncture is so effective in the treatment of many neurological disorders like epilepsy, muscular weakness, strokes, and facial paralysis.

The Homoeostatic Effect. The most important effect of acupuncture is the Homoeostatic Effect: that is, it restores the body's internal environment to its normal state. Acupuncture normalizes the rate of breathing, heart rate, blood pressure, metabolic rate, body temperature, and other vital body parameters. These functions are controlled by the brain through the secretion of various hormones. The net effect of the treatment is to restore the body to its normal state and maintain it in that state. Thus in a patient with high blood pressure, acupuncture restores the blood pressure to normal by restoring the hormonal balance. Further treatment helps to maintain the normal blood pressure. There is no possibility of excess of treatment causing low blood pressure, unlike with the use of drugs.

This homoeostatic effect is used to treat many diseases, including hormonal imbalances and hypertension and makes acupuncture a remarkably safe form of treatment with no side-effects.

Strengthens Immunity, Fights Infections. Acupuncture improves and stimulates the body's immunity by increasing the number of white blood cells, antibodies, and gamma globulins which fight infections in the blood. In acute infections, the prolonged use of antibiotic therapy can be considerably reduced by concurrent use of acupuncture. In chronic infections like bronchitis and sinusitis, acupuncture alone is very useful in curing the infection. In chronic sinusitis, when fibrosis around the sinus prevents antibiotics from penetrating adequately into the sinus, acupuncture treatment for 10-14 days can clear up the infection, prompt sinus drainage, and help the fibrosis to dissolve.

Regulates Physiological and Psychological Functions of the Brain. The soothing or calming effect of acupuncture is well-accepted and this is one of the reasons why acupuncture is so effective in the treatment of anxiety, insomnia, addictions, and mental disorders. Since acupuncture is able to normalize the secretion of various neurotransmitters, it is able to regulate the physiological and psychological functioning of the brain.

As Local Anaesthesia. Acupuncture induces analgesia, which means absence of pain. This principle is used to desensitize the patient against pain and the patient remains entirely conscious even during surgery.

Acupuncture anaesthesia is a simple procedure involving insertion of needles at specific acu-points and stimulating them with a needle stimulator*. The patient temporarily loses the ability to feel pain in the area where the operation is to be performed. It is a safe, effective, and easy-to-use method and is ideal for use in elderly people for whom any form of surgical anaesthesia is risky.

The other advantage of acupuncture anaesthesia is that the patient does not suffer from any post-operative dizziness, nausea, abdominal distension, or any other side-effects. The patient is up and about soon after the operation. He can eat food immediately and recovers very quickly as compared to the conventional forms of anaesthesia.

Acupuncture anaesthesia has been used to give analgesia for many types of operations of the chest, neck, and head. It has been successfully used in tonsillectomy, extraction of teeth, cataract surgery, operations of the skull and brain, thyroid surgery, lung biopsies, and open

---

* An electrical device from which leads are clipped onto the acupuncture needles.

Tonifying and Sedating: How Acupuncture Works?

Recently science has determined that human beings are complex bioelectric systems. This understanding has been the foundation of acupuncture practice for several thousand years. Energy circulates throughout the body along well-defined pathways. Points on the skin along these pathways are energetically connected to specific organs, body structures, and systems. If this energy circulation is disrupted, optimum function is affected, and this results in pain or illness.

Much of acupuncture is concerned with restoring free movement and the proper direction of such movement. Implicit in this approach is that illness cannot take root if there is vitality, harmony, and free movement of *Qi*. Conversely, disease takes root if *Qi* cannot circulate freely, or gets blocked, or there is excess of it. Acupuncture heals by increasing the vitality, that is, by tonifying, where required, or by reducing the excess *Qi*, that is, by sedating, where required. This is achieved by needling and stimulating the different acupuncture points.

Tonifying is applied in deficiency-type disturbances such as dizziness, low blood pressure, deficiency of body fluids, etc. It is characterized by careful needling in the direction of flow of *Qi* in the channels and long retention of needles. Slow insertion and quick withdrawal of needles is tonifying. Gentle manipulation of needles is essential. Moxibustion is another major tonifying method.

Sedating is applied in excess-type disturbances such as cramps, acute pain, hypertension, increased muscle tone, and increased secretion of body fluids. To achieve this, needles are manipulated vigorously following insertion against the direction of flow of *Qi* in the channels. The retention period is short. Quick insertion followed by a slow withdrawal is sedating. Intensive manipulation of needles is important for sedating.

heart surgery. Acupuncture anaesthesia has also been successfully employed for painfree childbirth. The use of acupuncture to aid childbirth reduces the pain of labour, and shortens the labour period by increasing the dilatation of the cervix. The patient feels comfortable and there is little or no pain. She is, therefore, in a position to cooperate, press down, and allow the child to be expelled quickly and smoothly.

Today, acupuncture anaesthesia is used widely across the world and has been refined into both a fine art and a science.

What Can Acupuncture Treat?

In acupuncture the approach is holistic and the symptoms or the condition is not isolated from the patient. And because it has a different diagnostic framework which is patient-centred, it is not appropriate to assess the effectiveness of acupuncture using the control or elimination of symptoms as a yardstick. Nevertheless, it is difficult to show the depth and scope of acupuncture's potential action without using this Western perspective and without giving examples in Western medical terms.

Thinking within a Western framework, therefore, the following types of illness — some of which are diseases, some disorders, and some symptoms — indicate the remarkably wide range of conditions which respond to treatment by acupuncture.

Conditions Which Respond to Acupuncture

Acidity
Acne
Alcoholism
Anal fissure
Angina pectoris
Anxiety
Appetite, excessive
Appetite, lack of
Athma, bronchial

Backache, low
Backache with or without sciatica
Baldness, patchy
Bedwetting in children
Behaviour disorders (not temperament) in children
Boils
Bronchitis

Caicaneal spur
Cancer pains
Cervicitis
Chest congestion
Cirrhosis of the liver
Colic, biliary & renal
Common cold
Conjunctivitis
Constipation
Convulsions, infantile
Cough, allergic
Cystitis

Depression
Diabetes mellitus
Diarrhoea
Dysentery

Earache
Eczema
Epilepsy

Fatigue
Fear of darkness
Flatulence
Frozen shoulder

Gastritis
Glaucoma
Goitre
Gynaecomastia

Hair loss
Headaches
Hematuria (passing blood in urine)
Hemiplegia (paralysis of one side of the body)
Hepatitis
Herpes
Hiccups
Hypertension (high blood pressure)
Hypogonadism

Hypotension (low blood pressure)
Hysteria

Impotence
Inability to learn at school
Indigestion
Insomnia
Irritable bowel syndrome

Laryngitis (hoarseness in voice)
Leucoderma
Leucorrhoea
Listlessness after chronic diseases

Masculinisation symptoms in women
Mastitis (see Pain in breasts)
Memory loss
Menopausal disorders
Menses, excessive bleeding
Menses, irregular
Menses, painful
Migraine
Muscular dystrophies
Myopia, early

Nausea
Nephritis
Nerve deafness
Neurasthenia
Night-blindness

Obesity
Oliguria (passing less urine)
Optic atrophy
Osteoarthritis of hip and knee joints

Pain in breasts (mastitis)
Pain in calf muscles
Pain in chest muscles
Pain in sole of foot
Palpitations
Pancreatitis
Paralysis in children
Paralysis, one side of the body
Parkinson's disease, early stages
Pelvic pain
Pimples
Polio
Poor memory in children
Post-operative weaknes
Premature ejaculation
Protatitis, early
Psoriasis

Retina, detached
Rheumatoid arthritis (pain in all joints)

Sinusitis
Sjogren's syndrome (rheumatoid arthritis and dryness of eyes)
Skin allergies
Slipped dissc (see Backache)
Smoking
Sneezing, allergic
Sore throat
Splenomegaly (enlargement of the spleen)
Spondylitis, ankylosing
Spondylitis, cervical
Squint
Stiff neck, acute
Sty
Sub-fertility
Substance abuse
Sweating, excessive

Tennis elbow
Tinnitus
Tonsillitis
Travel sickness
Trigeminal neuralgia (intense pain of the face)

Ulcerative colitis
Ulcers, chronic skin
Ulcers, duodenal
Ulcers, gastric
Ulcers, peptic
Urethritis
Urticaria (itching)

Vaginitis
Vertigo
Vitiligo
Vomiting

Whooping cough
Wounds, non-healing
Writer's cramps

Yawning, excessive

International Acceptance and Support

The World Health Organization, the medical branch of the United Nations, issued a provisional list of 41 diseases amenable to acupuncture treatment. These include respiratory ailments, pain and chronic pain conditions, Premenstrual Syndrome (PMS) and other gynaecological disorders, gastro-intestinal disorders, and many other health problems. These are mentioned below:

Respiratory Tract Disorders. Acute sinusitis, acute rhinitis, common cold, acute tonsillitis.

Bronco-Pulmonary Disorders. Acute bronchitis, bronchial asthma (most effective in children and in patients without associated diseases).

Eye Disorders. Acute conjunctivitis, central retinitis, myopia in children, optic nerve atrophy.

Mouth Cavity Disorders. Toothache, pain after tooth extraction, gingivitis, acute and chronic pharyngitis.

Gastro-Intestinal Disorders. Spasms of the oesophagus, hiccups, acute and chronic gastritis, hyperacidity, chronic duodenal ulcer, acute and chronic colitis, constipation, diarrhoea.

Gynaecological Disorders. Cervicitis, leucorrhoea, painful periods, irregular menses.

Neurological and Orthopaedic Disorders. Headaches, migraines, trigeminal neuralgia, facial paralysis, peripheral neuropathy, post-polio paralysis, nocturnal enuresis, intercostal neuralgia, periarthritis, tennis elbow, backaches, sciatica, rheumatoid arthritis, osteoarthritis, early cases of hemiplegia.

Frequency of Treatment

The course of treatment is decided after analysing each individual's requirements so that he receives the maximum benefit from the treatment.

It is a common practice to treat a patient daily until he starts to improve. The frequency of treatment is then reduced to three times a week, then twice a week, and finally, to once a week. The patient is asked to return for reassessment four weeks after the completion of treatment. This advise is often ignored by the patient who sees no reason to return to the acupuncturist when he is feeling well. This short-sighted attitude may lead to recurrence of the problem later.

Most patients have multiple problems that are interrelated. Acupuncture takes a holistic approach, attending to all the ailments of the patient. Even though there are

> **Does Acupuncture Hurt?**
>
> The question 'does it hurt?' is asked frequently by people seeking acupuncture treatment for the first time. The fear arises out of the natural instinct to protect oneself against any pain. On the one hand, some patients show very little sensitivity to the needles, and do not feel pain when needles are inserted. On the other hand, there may be increased sensitivity in particular areas or on particular meridians, relating to an energy imbalance. Further, a patient may feel more sensitive to the needles on one occasion than on another. In general, however, treatment is not painful, and when needling sensation occurs it does not last more than a few seconds. Most acupuncturists tend to develop their own needling technique to achieve effective treatment and minimum pain.

numerous incidences of quick and miraculous cures, some ailments respond slower than others. The patient should not feel disheartened if he finds that some of his problems take longer to get cured than others. A cure requires a balancing of the energy flow and may be a slow process. In long-standing ailments, the response to treatment is slow, as the energy flows that have been disturbed for many years can and do take time to return to normal.

Precautions

Acupuncture is a safe method of treatment with no side-effects when general precautions are observed. Nevertheless, complications can occur.

During acupuncture treatment, fainting may occur in nervous, tense, or tired patients. When acupuncture is performed with the patient in a sitting position, fainting is the most common complication and is seen in about 5-10 per cent of cases. To avoid this, patients are almost always treated while lying down.

During insertion of the needles, pain can occur due to clumsy insertion or blunt needles. If a patient moves during acupuncture treatment, this can cause pain. Therefore, the patient should be in a stable position. Tense or anxious patients feel more pain. However, by using special inserters for needle insertion, acupuncture has been made a totally painless treatment.

It is worth repeating that since acupuncture is a comprehensive system of preventive health care and health maintenance based on promoting the body's natural healing abilities, most conditions can be corrected or improved. The effectiveness of acupuncture is now well-documented and extends far beyond the popular belief that it is useful only in chronic pain management or as an analgesic.

5

Needles Used in Acupuncture

As mentioned earlier the word acupuncture is derived from two Latin words: *acus,* meaning 'needle', and *puncture,* meaning 'to penetrate'. The word acupuncture, therefore, means to penetrate with a needle. In ancient times, sharpened fish bones, bamboo sticks, and pointed stones were used to stimulate acupuncture points. However with the discovery of metal and development of techniques to mould it into different forms, metallic needles have replaced the earlier rather primitive tools. Today, very thin, hair-like needles are used to reach and stimulate the acupuncture points.

Types of Needles

The different kinds of needles in use are filiform stainless steel needles, embedding needles, plum blossom needles, hot needles, and prismatic needles. These are described in detail. Some practitioners sometimes prefer to use needles with gold and silver handles for their tonification and sedation properties respectively.

Filiform Stainless Steel Needles. The needles ordinarily used in acupuncture are filiform stainless steel needles. The steel used is flexible and unbreakable. The diameter of the needles varies from 0.2 to 0.6 mm and is often given as the gauge* 26-32, and the length of the needles varies from 12 mm to 102 mm. The needle consists of three parts: a tip, the body, and a handle. Generally needles of 25 mm to 38 mm length with a gauge of 30-32 are preferred. Thinner needles are used in children where minimal stimulation is required, while thicker needles are used for stronger stimulation. Longer needles are used for areas like the buttocks where the muscle mass is thick.

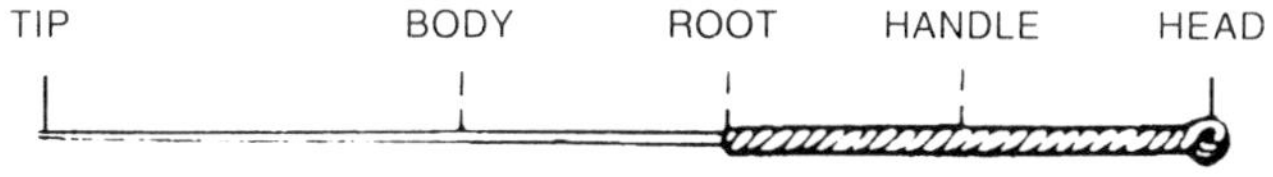

Fig. 7. Structure of the Filiform Needle

Embedding Needles. These needles are also called press needles, intradermal needles, or implanted needles. Embedding needles are inserted and left *in situ* (in their original place).

There are two types of embedding needles: thumbtack type and grain-like type. The commonest type are the thumbtack type, which are 2-3 mm long and have a small circular head at right angles to the shaft. They are most frequently used for ear acupuncture and may be pressed from time to time. Other designs of embedding needles, such as the grain-like type which are longer

* A standard measure for measuring thickness of metal.

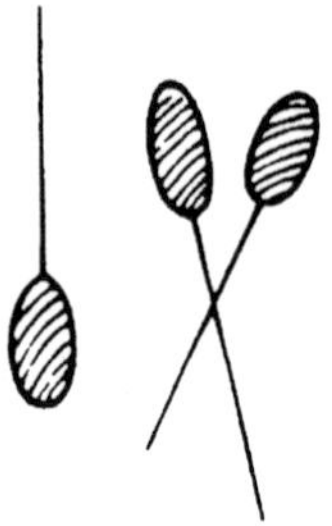

Fig. 8. Grain-like Type
Embedding Needles

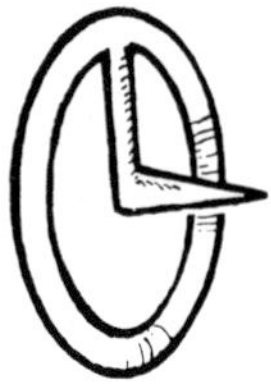

Fig. 9. Thumbtack Type
Embedding Needle

than the thumbtack type, are used for embedding at the other acupuncture points of the body.

Plum Blossom Needles. Another name for the plum blossom needles is seven star needles. These needles consist of seven short needles protruding out from a holder which is attached to a long handle. The instrument is used to tap along the meridians or on specific areas of the skin and is used in children, weak or elderly patients, or patients who dislike needles.

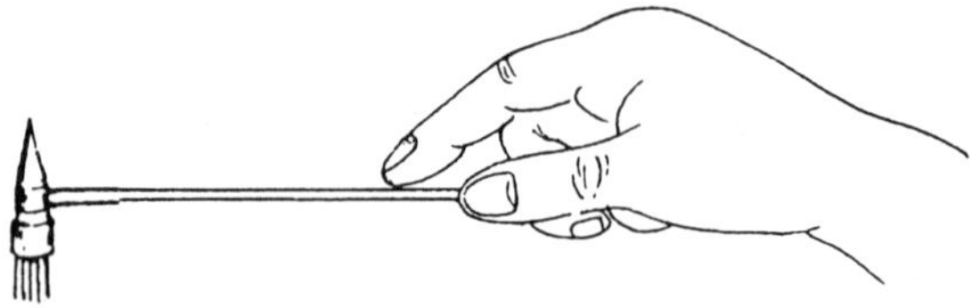

Fig. 10. Plum Blossom Needle

Hot Needles. Being fairly thick gauge needles, hot needles are made from a special alloy of silver. They are brought to red heat and plunged into certain types of superficial swellings and ganglions. The needles are withdrawn almost immediately so that they only remain in contact with the skin for a fraction of a second.

Prismatic Needles. Prismatic needles have triangular points. They are mostly used for certain types of inflammatory conditions, acute diseases, and allergic skin disturbances.

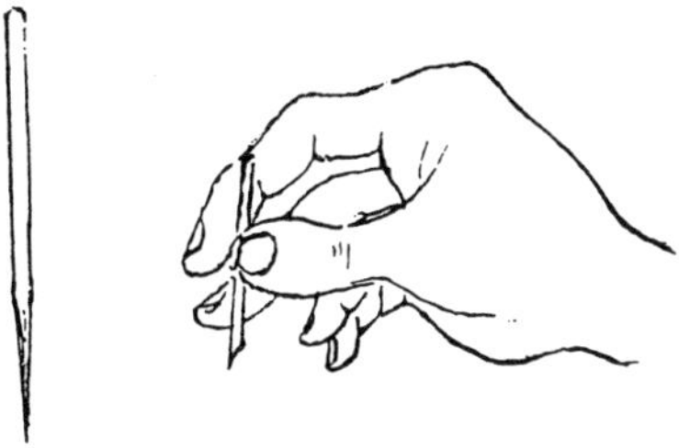

Fig. 11. A Prismatic Needle

Sterilization of Needles

There are established and strict procedures for needle sterilization. Acupuncture needles are generally sterilized in an autoclave, especially due to danger of contamination with the hepatitis and AIDS' viruses. Needles are sterilized with utmost care, and the exact time and temperature during sterilization is carefully controlled.

Simple disinfection or boiling of needles is totally inadequate. Needles tend to become blunt if used repeatedly. This leads to the treatment being more painful than it should be. Pre-sterilized, disposable needles are being increasingly used.

6

Traditional Acupuncture Techniques

Traditional Chinese Medicine (TCM) provides us with a complete explanation of how the body works, how the vital forces are formed, and how they may become unbalanced. Above all, it views the human body as a vital whole, infused with energy, which is more than the sum of the workings of its various organs. This, of course, is unlike the more mechanical view of Western medicine which sees the organism in purely physical terms. The practice of acupuncture with needles is an ancient technique. The balance and flow of energy is influenced by the insertion of fine needles into the acupuncture points, dispersing where there is excess, acting as a tonic in deficiency, cooling in heat, warming in cold, moving in stagnation, calming in agitation. It is a practical system to restore body harmony.

Acupuncturists do not just push needles into bodies in the way that doctors and nurses give hypodermic injections. Apart from the fact that the points, which are less than a millimetre each in diameter, have to be carefully located, the angle and depth of insertion vary at each point and have to be correctly observed. Some points are needled perpendicularly to the skin surface; many are needled at an angle of about 45 degrees; and some are needled almost horizontally with the needle making an angle of 15 to 25 degrees with the skin. In children the depth of insertion is significantly less than in adults. Needles can be inserted with the patient lying supine or prone, lateral, or sitting in a lithotomy* position.

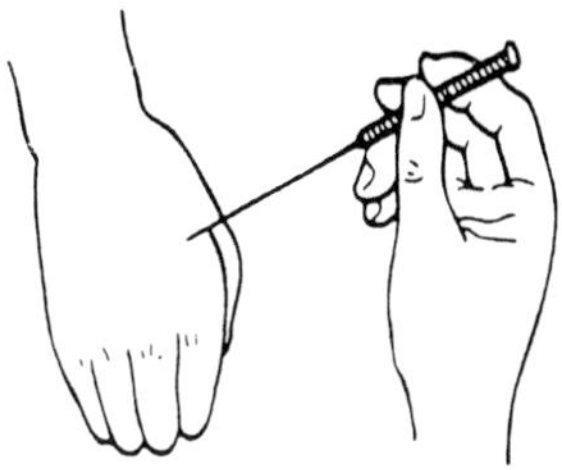

Fig. 12. Holding the Needle

Needles are inserted rapidly through the outer layers of tissue in order to make the operation as painless as poss·ble. From then onwards, the way in which the needle is introduced depends upon the type of treatment desired. In any event the acupuncturist aims to obtain a sensation felt by the patient which is

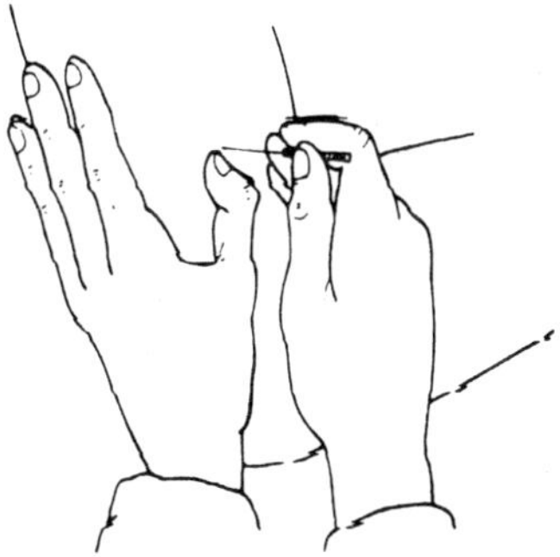

Fig. 13. Needle Insertion and Pressure Applied by the Other Hand

* Position assumed for the surgical removal of a stone from the urinary tract, especially the bladder.

termed as *de qi**. This is a sensation of numbness, tingling, heaviness, soreness, distension, or a feeling of slight pain at a distance from the site of puncture. Frequently, *de qi* is felt as a radiating sensation and experienced along the acupuncture meridian.

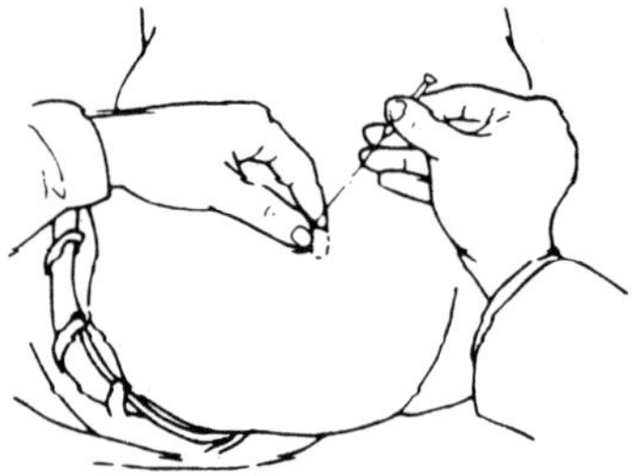

Fig. 14. Inserting the Needle by Coordinating the Puncturing and Pressing Hands

Different qualities of *de qi* are usually obtained in different areas. Where the muscle mass is thin, the feeling is usually that of local distension, whereas if the muscle is thick, it is usually one of numbness or soreness. If the acupuncture point is close to a nerve trunk, the sensation is likely to be that of tingling or 'electric shock'. In some instances *de qi* cannot be obtained and this does not mean that the treatment is not working. It must be stressed that *de qi*, although not pleasant, is quite distinct from the sensation of pain.

De qi may also be picked up by the acupuncturist and is recognizable as a sense of tightening felt through the needle handle which results from local muscle spasm in the patient. Some acupuncturists claim to be able to feel a subtle sensation on the hand during needling.

Manipulation of Needles

Manipulation of needles is essential for a tonifying (enhancing) or sedating (suppressing) effect on energy.

---

* The sensation felt by the acupuncturist or the patient or both when the tip of the needle touches the nerve ending at the precise acupuncture point.

If the treatment is for local pain or stagnation (blockage of energy flow), it will be more necessary to manipulate the needles, whereas treatment to balance the patient's energies will require very little manipulation, as correct insertion will ensure the required effect. The needles may be manipulated in one of the following ways:

- Lifting and thrusting
- Rotation — clockwise and counter-clockwise
- Combination of rotation with lifting and thrusting

Thrusting Technique. In this technique the needle is thrust up and down by a push-pull force exerted on the handle. The correct depth is first obtained through *de qi* and the needle then lifted just a few millimetres and immediately returned to the original depth. The amplitude of the movement is increased for very strong stimulation, but the needle is by no account completely withdrawn. If *de qi* is not obtained the angle of the return thrust is varied slightly with a view to seek the depth at which *de qi* exists. (see Fig. 15).

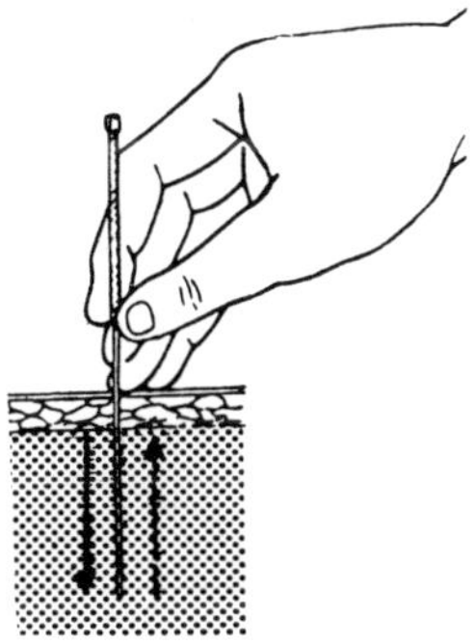

Fig. 15. Thrusting Technique

Twirling Technique. In this case the needle is introduced to the correct depth and then rotated almost 180 degrees. This is usually repeated for about half a minute, allowing the needle to return to neutral more or less by itself. According to tradition, if the needle is rotated clockwise, it invokes a stimulating process (tonifying) and if anti-clockwise, it causes sedation (see Fig. 16).

Combination Techniques. This is a more difficult manoeuvre to perform but generally gives better results. It is also thought that by thrusting the needle when the patient is breathing out and raising or lifting during inspiration, a greater degree of stimulation (tonifying) is obtained and, conversely, by introducing the needle during the inspiratory phase and withdrawing it during expiration, a greater degree of sedation is brought about. Manual manipulation has to be done fairly rapidly and has to be sustained for the duration of the entire treatment.

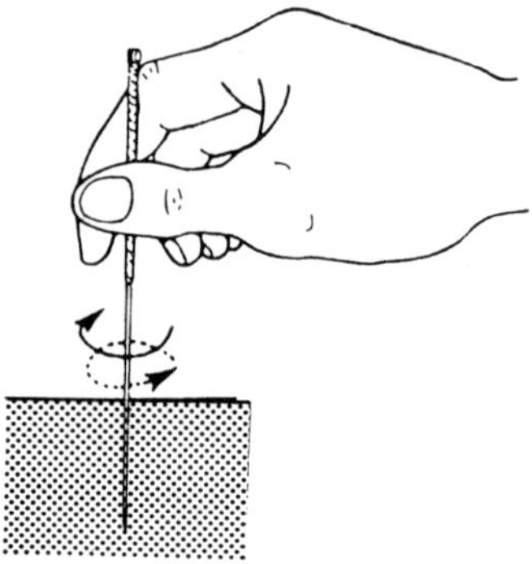

Fig. 16. Twirling Technique

7

Non-Traditional Acupuncture Techniques

While the practice of acupuncture with needles is the traditional technique (see chapter 6), significant research and experimentation in modern times has modified it to suit specific and special therapeutic requirements.

Some of the common methods being used in acupuncture today are electro-acupuncture, aquapuncture, homoeo-puncture, catgut-embedding therapy, point injection therapy, bleeding technique, auto-immunization therapy, skin-embedded needle therapy, and scalp acupuncture.

Electro-Acupuncture. Electro-acupuncture is a technique which was developed in the mid-nineteenth century. Le Chevalier Sarlandiere was the first to apply electric stimulation to the implanted needles. In 1825 he reported cures in asthma, paralysis, migraine, and rheumatism. Two other French physicians, Jules Coquet and T.M. Dantu, described the treatment of many kinds of intractable pain including facial neuralgia with electro-acupuncture. They sometimes left the needles in for as long as eight hours though they also reported near instantaneous relief of pain.

It has been found that efficacy of acupuncture is greatly enhanced by electrical stimulation and for several decades many doctors have reported enhanced analgesic and therapeutic effects with different kinds of electrical stimulation. China has been foremost in conducting these experiments. In China, surgery under acupuncture analgesia was first performed in 1960s using electro-acupuncture. In this technique, manual manipulation of needles was replaced by stimulation of the acupuncture points by vibrating the needles, with a weak, controlled current generated through a stimulator. The electro-stimulators are generally battery-operated and stimulation is regulated according to the tolerance and comfort of the patient. Electrical stimulation used is more reliable, less tiring, and more acceptable to the patient.

Higher frequencies are used for surgical analgesia but lower frequencies are normally employed for routine acupuncture. Today electro-acupuncture is very popular all over the world, including China, particularly for treatment of acute conditions. Most electro-stimulators in use are fitted with a point detector to locate the correct points which often lie so close to each other that it is difficult to locate the exact point manually.

Precautions: Electro-acupuncture should not be used for young children, very old persons, epileptic patients or those in other convulsive conditions, mentally deranged patients, and patients suffering from shock, fever, restlessness, and over-anxiety.

Aquapuncture. In this particular form of acupuncture a small volume of fluid — usually a vitamin solution or distilled water — is injected into the site of the acupuncture point. The rationale is to stimulate micro-circulation (circulation in the finer blood vessels near the surface of the skin) in that area, which in turn promotes healing.

Homoeopuncture. Homoeopuncture is a new technique in which homoeopathy is combined with acupuncture. The acupuncture needle is dipped into the liquid form of the homoeopathic medicine prescribed for a patient by a homoeopath and is inserted at a specific acupuncture point. Since a specific remedy for a specific disease is inserted directly into the tissue, it acts immediately and enhances its effect. Initial results appear to be encouraging, but it requires further research, trials, and observations before it can be confidently asserted that these two different therapies can be used and administered together.

Catgut-Embedding Therapy. This is a technique in which a surgical catgut suture is embedded at an acupuncture point with the aim of giving constant stimulation to the point.

In this treatment a needle with catgut is inserted at a specific acupuncture point. The needle is then withdrawn leaving the catgut embedded in the skin. This catgut is left in position for a period of 3 to 4 weeks till it dissolves on its own. During the time that the catgut is embedded, it gives constant stimulation to the acupuncture point and helps in achieving quicker results.

This therapy is particularly useful in resistant cases of chronic bronchial asthma, chronic backaches, post-polio paralysis, traumatic paraplegia, cerebrovascular accidents (strokes) with hemiplegia, and chronic hyperacidity.

Point Injection Therapy. This therapy is a combination of Western medicine and traditional medicine. In this method a small amount of therapeutic medicine, prescribed according to the principles of, and by a qualified practitioner of Western medicine, is injected at the acupuncture points. This works by stimulating the micro-circulation and increasing the body resistance, thus helping in the curative effect.

Drugs used for this therapy include vitamins B_1, B_2, B_6, and B_{12}, and distilled water. Treatment is given once daily or on alternate days for 6-7 days, and repeated after a gap of 7-10 days, if necessary. Point injection therapy is especially recommended for asthma, lumbago, allergies, skin disorders, and other painful conditions.

Bleeding Technique. The bleeding technique is performed by puncturing certain specific acupuncture points and bringing out one or two drops of blood to remove the stagnation in the blood. This is specifically useful in chronic skin diseases, as also in emergencies like coma, convulsions, and stroke.

Auto-Immunization Therapy. In this form of therapy, a drop of blood from one acupuncture point is taken out and injected into another acupuncture point. This therapy has been found to be a useful add-on in the treatment of all types of allergic diseases, particularly in allergic bronchial asthma, allergic rhinitis and sinusitis, skin diseases like chronic eczema, psoriasis, and dermatitis, skin rashes, and itching.

Skin-Embedding Needle Therapy. Skin-embedding needles which are slightly longer and whose shaft lies in the same plane as the body are used at certain body acupuncture points for continuous stimulation for a few days. They are effective in treating very intractable painful conditions.

Micro-Acupuncture Systems

Therapeutic systems similar to micro-acupuncture systems have been practised since ancient times without the practitioners being aware of the principles behind their healing effects in various diseases. It has now been found that the effectiveness of these systems is based on the fact that small areas of the human body like the ears, scalp, hands, and feet have acupuncture points representing all the organs of the body. These systems are additional tools for an acupuncturist to achieve a better effect in a particular disease. They are used as complementary to the main system of acupuncture and never or seldom used independently.

Ear Acupuncture. Ear acupuncture or auriculotherapy is that branch of acupuncture which makes use of the external ear to diagnose as well as to treat illnesses. This form of treatment has been widely practised in different parts of the world. In older times physicians cauterized the ear with a red hot poker to treat sciatica. Ayurvedic practitioners in ancient India inserted earrings into various parts of the ear to treat diseases like asthma and arthritis. The practice of wearing earrings was not merely ornamental but often had a therapeutic purpose as well.

Recently a great deal of work on ear acupuncture has been done by Dr Paul Nogier of France, which

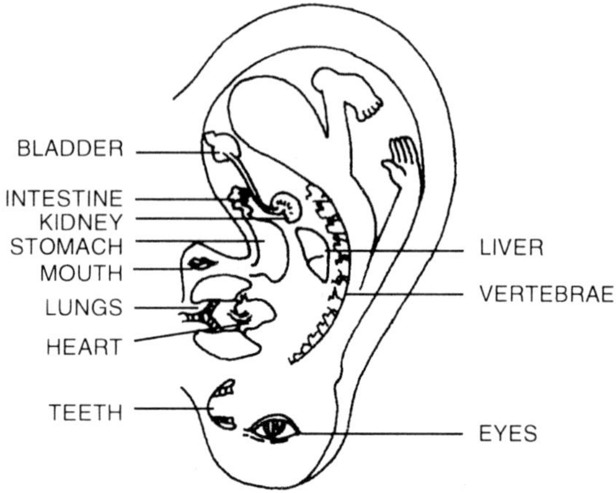

Fig. 17. Ear Acupuncture. *The outer ear is in the shape of an upside-down foetus.*

has lead to the proliferation of this form of therapy in Europe. The ear is said to contain 136 acupuncture points which are arranged in the ear in the form of an upside-down foetus. The head is represented at the lobule of the ear, while the feet lie at the top of the ear. The other organs are distributed through the other parts of the ear. The principle behind ear acupuncture is that when a point in the ear is stimulated, it creates an effect on the corresponding organ.

In this form of acupuncture, small needles are inserted and stimulated by hand or with a high frequency electric current. Where prolonged stimulation of an acupuncture point is required, as in certain internal organ disorders, a small ear-press needle is left *in situ* (in its original place) for a period of 7 to 10 days to obtain a better response. The ear-press needles are circular in form, and about 3 mm in diameter with a tip which penetrates to a depth of 2-3 mm. These are left in position with an adhesive tape.

The insertion of needles in the ear is used to treat a range of conditions including anxiety, insomnia, epilepsy, hypertension, hormonal imbalances, and pain due to many causes. Ear acupuncture has also been used to help overweight people to slim down. Whenever the person feels an urge to eat, he is advised to place his thumb and forefinger on either side of the ear and massage the needle. This process releases neurotransmitters in the brain which takes away the urge to eat by making the stomach feel full.

Ear acupuncture is also useful in helping people to quit smoking. The treatment effectively counteracts the effect of nicotine withdrawal. It removes the physical need to smoke and many patients develop an aversion to cigarettes. This is achieved by stimulating the nicotine receptors in the brain, so that the patient does not manifest any physical signs of withdrawal. Whenever the patient feels the urge to smoke, he is advised to massage the ear-press needle — this removes the urge. The smoker needs to be cautioned that he should not light a cigarette out of habit and should have the will to stop smoking.

Ear acupuncture is also helpful in treating drug addiction. The patient experiences very few withdrawal symptoms and is easily able to give up the habit, provided he has the will to quit the use of drugs.

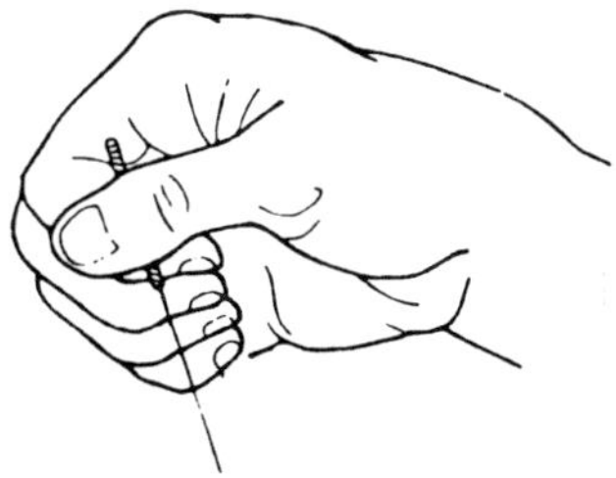

Fig. 18. Holding the Needle for Scalp Acupuncture

Scalp Acupuncture. This form of acupuncture has come into use lately. In this type of acupuncture, fine acupuncture needles are inserted at specific areas of the scalp and left for a period of twenty minutes. The main indications for scalp acupuncture are hemiplegia, paraplegia, complications following cerebrovascular accidents, hypertension, trembling of hands and early stages of Parkinson's disease, certain vision disturbances, vertigo, ringing in the ears, deafness, speech problems, impotence, neurosis, bedwetting in children, bronchial asthma, gastric ulcers, and gynaecological and urinary disorders (see Figs. 18 and 19). It is used along with body acupuncture.

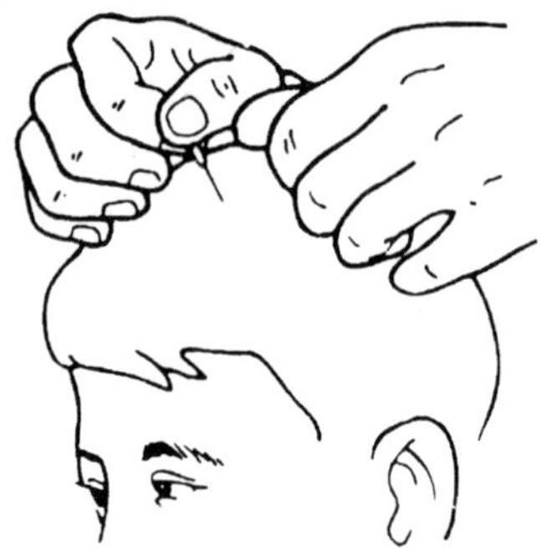
Fig. 19. Rotating the Needle for Scalp Acupuncture

Hand Acupuncture. Hand acupuncture involves inserting needles at acupuncture points in the hands to cure various diseases. Around 200 BC, it was written in *The Yellow Emperor's Classic of Internal Medicine* that stimulating acupuncture points in the hands by needles adjusts the balance between *Yin* and *Yang* and, therefore, cures sickness. There are altogether 36 regular acupuncture points found in the hands, 20 on the dorsal surface (back) of the hands and 16 on the palmar surface (front) of the hands. In addition, there are 6 extra points which are commonly used, 3 on the palmar surface and 3 on the dorsal surface. Hand acupuncture is especially good for acute pain. However for chronic illnesses, certain specific acupuncture points on the dorsal and palmar surface of the hands are needled along with the body, ear, or scalp acupuncture points to achieve better results. (see Figs. 20 and 21).

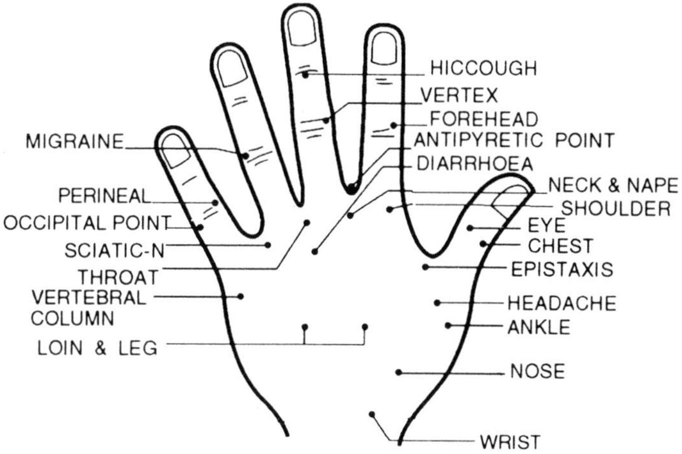

Fig. 20. Points Used in Hand Acupuncture (Dorsal Surface)

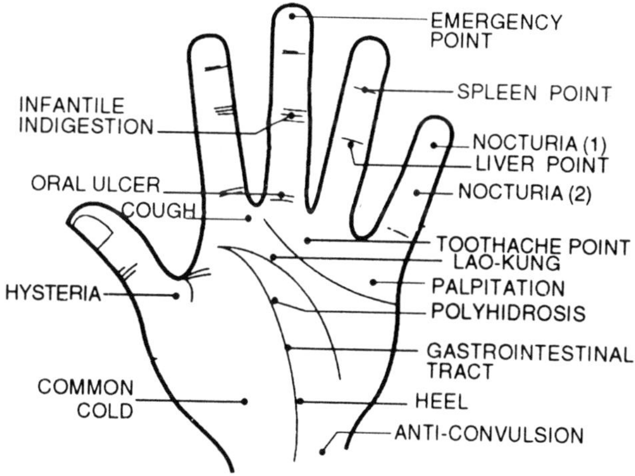

Fig. 21. Points Used in Hand Acupuncture (Palmar Surface)

Wrist and Ankle Acupuncture. This group of acupuncture points has been found to be very effective in treating acute painful disorders, rhinitis, asthma, and insomnia.

Nose and Face Acupuncture. This is a very specialised technique in which very fine cosmetic needles are inserted in the area of the nose and face. This can be combined with body, ear, and scalp acupuncture.

Periosteal Acupuncture. This method of treatment was discovered by Dr Felix Mann of UK in 1974 and it was first mentioned by him in the third edition of his book entitled *Treatment of Disease by Acupuncture.* It employs lifting and thrusting of a needle to stimulate an acupuncture point. However it differs from other forms of acupuncture in that the needle is lifted and pressed down till it touches the covering of the bone. This lifting and thrusting is repeated for some time. The treatment is particularly useful in resistant cases of pain in the joints where routine acupuncture therapy does not produce the desired relief. It is mainly indicated in arthritis of the knee, elbow, and shoulder joints, hip joint pains, pain in the small joints of the hands and feet, and pain in the spinal column.

8

Scientific Techniques in Acupuncture

In spite of the huge amount of money spent on research, development, and practice of Western medicine, many practising doctors and even more patients are dissatisfied with modern Western medicine. It is widely acknowledged that the Western medical system has several shortcomings including adverse effects of drugs administered.

Development and application of modern scientific techniques has given acupuncture a big advantage of early diagnosis. An early diagnosis not only means finding a problem at the early stage of imbalance of energy, before this imbalance leads to serious adverse effects on the body and mind, but also leads to better and healthier living. Early diagnosis and preventive medicine are not possible until the electromagnetic energy field and the electric energy pathways of the body are tapped for information.

The electro-dermal diagnosis (checking the electro-conductivity at an acupuncture point located under the dermis) of the human body based on testing the electrical state of acupuncture points, holds the promise of being a faster, cheaper, and a more accurate method of early diagnosis than the present chemical, analytic, and photo-imaging methods.

Much research has been done in Japan, Germany, Australia, USA, and other countries to compare the electro-diagnostic measurement of acu-points with various medical syndromes, signs, symptoms, and diseases. The recent introduction of advanced computer technology into electro-acupuncture diagnosis has further improved both reliability and ease of diagnosis.

Ryodoraku: The Japanese Contribution to Acupuncture

Ryodoraku electro-acupuncture is an electro-diagnostic and stimulatory technique based on the theories of classical acupuncture. It represents a significant step forward from classical acupuncture as it allows the subjective traditional diagnosis to be substituted by mechanical recording of energy deficiency/excess in various channels. It was developed after many years of research and observations of electric current recordings made over acupuncture points.

These readings were analysed and representative measurement points on each acupuncture channel were charted. The readings of the electro-conductivity over the 24 representative measurement points (RMPs) were recorded on the *Ryodoraku* graph. When we use a *Ryodoraku* graph it shows the relative state of homoeostatic balance between the twelve body channels and organs and gives us useful principles for treatment.

When the readings over all RMPs are within the normal range, then all the channels and organs are said to be well-balanced and healthy. Channels where the readings are below the normal range, are tonified, and those with readings above the normal range, are sedated. If the measured values are outside of the normal physiological range and the associated symptoms are not present, it suggests that the patient is manifesting a new symptom or the patient has had an illness in the past and is in the process of recovery.

After appropriate treatment, deviations from the normal physiological range are gradually diminished and the various signs and symptoms get relieved.

Acutech

Acutech is a modern computerised version of the popular Japanese scientific acupuncture known as *Ryodoraku* or the Autonomous Nerve Regulatory Therapy.

How Acutech Works? In it a probe is used to measure the energy flow of 12 acu-points (point of maximum energy flow in each of the 12 channels) bilaterally on the hands and feet. Through these points the channels and organs in the body can be tested for electrical imbalance. An electrical imbalance is a sign of a disease or pre-disease state. The pre-disease state is an early stage and can usually be quickly reversed.

Through these remarkable advances in electro-acupuncture diagnosis, we can detect and treat diseases while they are in the electrical imbalance stage (pre-symptom stage) rather than after cellular changes have taken place. In most cases when sufficient cellular changes have taken place to make a disease visible through testing procedures, it is usually difficult or impossible to reverse the condition. However, at the stage of an electrical imbalance, we can reverse the condition even before the symptoms appear. This is, in actuality, preventive medicine, and as such should be the very essence of medical practice, irrespective of the modality of treatment used by the practitioner.

With this equipment, it is also possible to locate tender points with high conductivity. The search for points with higher conductivity is carried out over the area where the patient is experiencing the problem, that is, the lower back in backaches, the chest in asthma, and the abdomen in colitis.

Acutech has a significant advantage over the classical method of diagnosis in acupuncture as it allows diagnosis to be made with accuracy, and the results of treatment can be scientifically monitored and evaluated.

Disorders Conducive to Acutech

Abdominal pains	Low back pain
Arthropathy	Menopausal problems
Autonomic nerve disorders	Migraine
Bronchial asthma	Muscular pains
Cervical spondylitis	Neuralgias
Enuresis	Osteoarthritis
Facial paralysis	Periarthritis
Headaches	Rheumatoid arthritis
Herpes zoster	Sciatica
Hypertension	Sprains
Insomnia	Stiff neck and shoulder
Knee pain	Tonsillitis
	Toothache

Our experience of using Acutech also supports that it provides greater objectivity in diagnosis and therefore the treatment becomes more accurate. This in turn leads to a higher success rate.

During 1996-99 we observed and recorded the success rate of Acutech based treatment on 150 patients treated at our clinic. The success rate was 100%, with some of the patients getting relief within 2 days of starting the treatment. What was notable was that 100% of the patients got relief.

Treated for 2 days	18%
Treated for 3-6 days	16%
Treated for 7 days	16%
Treated for 10 days and above	50%

We use this modern diagnostic tool frequently in our practice.

9

Needleless Acupuncture

Energy flows through the meridians. Acupuncture influences this energy flow by needling the acupuncture points which lie along these meridians to achieve a harmonious balance between physical, emotional, and spiritual states. Of late, the same effect has been achieved without the use of needles. These needleless techniques offer the advantage of being non-invasive and, therefore, non-traumatic. Individuals who are scared of needles have an intuitive preference for such techniques, as also children, the frail, and the elderly. Being non-invasive there is no risk of infection or bruise. These techniques are also used for self-acupuncture and for cosmetic use.

Transcutaneous Electro-Acupuncture

Transcutaneous electro-acupuncture is a mode of treatment wherein electrodes made of rubber or metal are placed on the skin over the acupuncture points. A battery powered micro-stimulator is used to pass a small electric current through the skin to stimulate the acupuncture points. As these conductive pads are fairly broad the electric current is picked up by sensitive acupuncture points.

The electrodes are fastened securely with an adhesive tape or an elastic band to ensure good contact between the skin and the electrode over the acupuncture points. The intensity control of the stimulator is slowly increased until the patient can just feel the stimulation. It is a sign of improvement when the intensity of the stimulation required in the same patient gradually reduces with the progress of the treatment. The efficacy of this treatment is directly related to the correct placement of the electrodes and the electrical contact between the electrodes and the skin. It is based on the principle that the electrical resistance of the skin over a sensitive acupuncture point is less as compared to the surrounding skin. So these acupuncture points will conduct electricity much better than the surrounding skin.

This treatment is more acceptable to patients who are apprehensive of needles but are willing to tolerate the slight discomfort associated with the flow of electrical impulses from the electrodes through their skin. This is an effective modality of treatment even though it is not as quick as traditional acupuncture with needles. It has the advantage in that the skin electrodes are reusable. It is useful in many common ailments like cold, sore throat, headache, insomnia, anxiety, constipation, fractures, sprains, and drug addiction. Very often the patient can be trained to treat himself and the availability of relatively inexpensive electro-acupuncture stimulators makes this a viable proposition.

Stipuncture:
Electrical Stimulation of Energy Points

Stipuncture is an electronic marvel which was invented in France. With this instrument, we can balance the flow of energy in our body. If a patient has a problem it could be the result of blocked, insufficient, or retarded energy in the region where the problem exists. If the circulation of energy is insufficient, stimulation is required; if energy is blocked, dispersion needs to be done. The instrument allows the detection of the exact location of the point to be stimulated. Each acupuncture point is electrically treated for 15 to 20 seconds to achieve the desired results. The simplicity and precision of the equipment guarantees quick and effective results.

Acutron

Acutron is a modern health care tool having several advantages over needle acupuncture. It is totally painless to the patient. It has various inbuilt programmes which utilize micro and interferential currents at acupuncture points to give quicker and long-lasting relief to the patient without inserting needles. It is used for pain management. The treatment proves to be effective in 70 to 80 per cent of the patients. Many painful conditions, particularly slipped disc, can be managed very well with acutron and surgery can be avoided. It also reduces the healing time in various medical conditions by 30 to 60 per cent.

Some specific conditions in which acutron is effective includes acute and chronic low back pain, neck and shoulder pain, sinus headaches, extremities and joint pains, sprains and strains, fibromyalgia, rheumatoid arthritis, and sports injuries. Acutron treatment can be highly effective in healing non union bone fractures. It accelerates the reduction of inflammation associated with bone fracture and muscle damage. It is also utilized to improve muscle power and correct muscle wasting in conditions like polio myelitis, paralysis, etc.

Laser Acupuncture

The therapeutic properties of light have been known for thousands of years. Human efforts to harness the power of light for healing reached its culmination with the development of *laser* — light amplification by stimulated emission of radiation. The essential characteristics of a laser beam are its unidirectional movement, single colour, and single focus. The laser beam has ushered in a new era in medicine due to the availability of pure beams of light of several different wavelengths. The therapeutic penetration of a laser depends upon its wavelength and availability of different wavelengths enhances its therapeutic potential.

In 1975, the first helium-neon laser device with a wavelength of 632 nm* was introduced in Germany. Later infra-red lasers with a 904 nm wavelength and 5-10 mw** intensity were developed. The latest developments are diode laser devices with a 780 nm wavelength and 10-30 mw intensity. These low-energy laser systems with intensity below 100 mw are also called soft lasers.

Laser is harmless since it is a pure and highly focussed beam of light. It is able to travel through the skin to stimulate the acupuncture points which are located

* One Nano Metre (nm) = One thousand millionth of a metre.
** One Milli Watt (mw) = One thousandth of a watt.

up to a depth of a centimeter below the skin's surface. When a laser is applied to the skin, most people do not feel any sensation, but some patients do feel a slight warmth, and a throbbing or tickling sensation.

Each acupuncture point is stimulated for 30-60 seconds. The duration of exposure at each acupuncture point is decided by the power of the laser. Thus, a 10 mw laser (infra-red or diode laser) requires a greater duration of exposure per point as compared to a 30 mw laser (diode laser), which requires less time per acupuncture point. In a busy acupuncture clinic, a 30 mw diode laser is likely to be used. Treatment with a laser may take longer as compared to conventional acupuncture since laser penetration is less than what can be achieved by manual insertion of needles. Lower level of penetration also means lesser degree of stimulation. If conventional acupuncture can treat a backache in 20 sittings, it will require about 30 sittings to achieve the same effect with laser acupuncture.

Helium-neon lasers were the first lasers to be used in acupuncture. These lasers generate a bright light at a wavelength of 632.8 nm. A helium-neon laser has a penetration of 2-3 mm and is best suited for the treatment of skin conditions. With its use, the skin is gradually tightened by improving the tone of the skin and the facial muscles and by improving blood supply to the area. The other conditions where the helium-neon laser produces dramatic results are facelifts, treating acne, scars, crow's feet, wrinkles, and skin diseases like eczema, herpes zoster, and psoriasis. It is also used in children and in a few other conditions where the acupuncture points lie close to the surface of the skin.

The infra-red lasers are used to stimulate acupuncture

points and are useful in the treatment of most chronic disorders which are amenable to acupuncture.

Sonopuncture (Ultrasound Puncture)

The term sonopuncture is used for acupuncture carried out by using a narrow, cylindrical, high-frequency beam of sound instead of needles. The human ear is capable of hearing sound waves between 20-20,000 cycles per second. Sound waves with a frequency of 20,000 cycles per second or more are too high pitched to be heard by the human ears and are called ultrasound. Ultrasound waves are obtained by applying an alternating electric current to the face of a quartz crystal, causing it to vibrate. High frequency sound waves of 750,000 to 1,000,000 cycles per second are most effective for sonopuncture.

Sound waves applied to the acupuncture meridian system have been found to be safe and effective, This method has an advantage over needle acupuncture in that it is totally painless and therefore has better patient acceptability.

For sonopuncture, specially constructed high quality sound heads are used that generate a narrow cylindrical beam of ultrasound. These special-purpose sound heads emit intense vertical beams ranging around 2-5 mm in width. Each of these special-purpose sound heads are handcrafted to exacting standards to ensure that the beam is uniform. Small sound heads are used to treat acupuncture points in children, medium to large-sized sound heads for adults, auricular sound heads to especially treat the ear acupuncture points, vaginal and rectal sound heads to treat local conditions in these areas, and special roller electrodes to give transcutaneous stimulation for pain control.

Sonopuncture is a quick method of therapy that requires 30-60 seconds of stimulation at each acupuncture point. It has an effective depth of penetration of 6-8 cm. This penetration is possible because ultrasound waves are conducted through fat without absorption and are absorbed by the underlying muscle where most acupuncture points are situated. This makes sonopuncture an effective alternative to acupuncture even in very fat patients.

While doing sonopuncture, a conducting medium like a gel or oil is required between the sound head and the skin to conduct ultrasound waves into the body. Without the gel the ultrasound waves are reflected inside the sound head, generating heat instead of helping the body to heal itself.

The effectiveness of sonopuncture in curing various diseases have been demonstrated by many workers in the field. The results of some of these studies carried out by Dr William H Khoe, MD in Las Vegas, USA, and published in the *American Journal of Acupuncture* (vol. 1, 1993) are given below:

Treatment of Infections. Sonopuncture is very effective in the treatment of infections where routine needle acupuncture does not work. Sonopuncture works by improving the blood circulation in the area being treated. There is an increase in the circulation of blood, which brings the white blood cells and antibodies to the affected area. This speeds up the process of healing in the treatment of small abscesses and non-healing wounds.

As a Cosmetic Aid. Sonopuncture is used in removing facial wrinkles and scars. Ageing and wrinkled skin gradually smoothens out and begins to glow again, while the underlying muscles become firm. It helps to improve the elasticity of scar tissue and is the treatment of choice following surgery to ensure a soft smooth scar.

For Varicose Veins. Sonopuncture is extremely useful in patients with varicose veins. It improves the tone of the affected veins — they start to contract and within 6-8 weeks, most patients respond adequately. However, chronic patients require 20 to 24 weeks of treatment.

For Spinal Problems. Sonopuncture is effective in providing almost immediate relief in many conditions like backaches, fibrositis, and ankylosing spondylitis. Strong stimulation is given at tender acupuncture points and in 3 to 5 minutes, the patient experiences relief. Ankylosing spondylitis, which is a crippling condition causing pain and stiffness of the entire spine, responds very well to sonopuncture.

Sports Medicine. Sonopuncture is used by athletes before a race to achieve peak physical performance. Sonopuncture is also very effective in treating bruises, ligament tears, and any other inflammation. Massaging the area speeds up the healing process. A sprain or a strain takes 3 to 6 weeks to heal, but with sonopuncture it can heal in 7 to 10 days. Thus this treatment is very useful in treating professional sportsmen as it permits an early return to complete physical fitness.

Quick Healing Fractures. Sonopuncture can also be used to promote healing of fractured bones. The time of healing of fractures can be reduced to half by the use of sonopuncture, and even fractures which have not healed for months can be persuaded to heal quickly.

Dental Ailments. Dental ailments are also helped by sonopuncture. Loose teeth can be made stronger by using sonopuncture for a few weeks. With this therapy, teeth which would have had to be extracted, can be saved and made healthy again. Sonopuncture is also useful in the treatment of inflammation of the gums, cavities, and tempromandibular joint (facial joint used in opening the mouth) pain.

Asthma and Bronchial Problems. Treatment with sonopuncture can provide immediate relief from bronchospasms in cases of asthma, thus making breathing easier in 5 to 10 minutes. It is also very useful in treating an enlarged prostate and benign nodular enlargement of the breast.

10

Su Jok Acupuncture

'*Su Jok*' is a Korean word meaning hand and foot. *Su Jok* acupuncture is a general term describing a new system of disease treatment, comprising a variety of methods of stimulating only the hands and feet with needles, moxa, stimulators, seeds, and lasers, or with the help of finger pressure therapy to effect a cure.

This new system of acupuncture was developed by Professor Park Jae Woo of Korea in the 1980s. After years of careful observations, research, and clinical experiences, he concluded that by stimulating points only on the hands and feet the entire body and all its systems could be healed. He published his findings in 1987 and founded the *Su Jok* (Hand and Foot) Acupuncture System.

The advantage of this system is its simplicity, safety, and efficiency. It is easy to learn and the speed of response is often dramatic. It contains no forbidden or dangerous points and is therefore also suitable for use by paramedics and lay persons for self-treatment.

How *Su Jok* Works?

The theoretical basis of this system is the discovery of a similar shape as of a human body on each hand and each foot. This miniature reflection of the human body also represents its structure, the systems, and the various organs, at a micro level. These micro-systems act as remote controls and can therefore be used easily to treat any diseased area or organ in the body. These are highly active points located on hands and feet and correspond to all the organs and parts of the body. Stimulation of these treatment points produces both a curative and a prophylactic effect.

The Hand and Foot Correspondence Systems. In the basic correspondence systems, the thumb corresponds to the head; the palm and sole, to the trunk; the third and fourth fingers and toes correspond to the legs; and the second and fifth fingers and toes correspond to the arms.

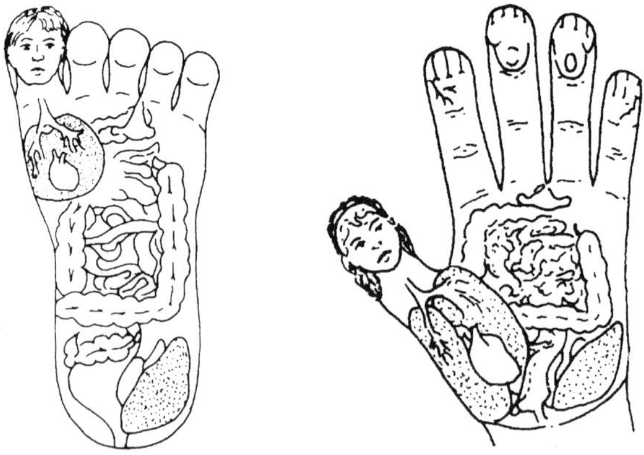

Fig. 22. Human Anatomy Represented on Hand and Foot.

The hand is positioned, palm front, to locate the points. The right hand's forefinger and left hand's little finger correspond to the right arm. The right hand's third finger and the left hand's fourth finger correspond to the right leg. The right hand's fourth finger and the left hand's third finger correspond to the left leg. The right hand's little finger and the left hand's forefinger correspond to the left arm. The elevated area on the palm, below the thumb, corresponds to the chest, and the palm as a whole corresponds to the abdominal region.

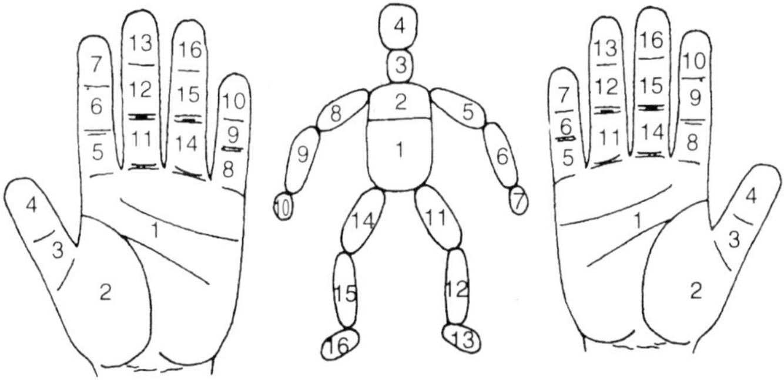

Fig. 23. Body Parts Represented on the Hands with Corresponding Numbers

The body and the corresponding micro-systems on hands and feet interact continuously. When an illness strikes, the affected organ or body part sends a 'signal' to its corresponding point, exciting it. The point turns painful. When this point is stimulated, a 'curing effect' springs up which normalizes the sick body part.

In *Su Jok* acupuncture, the response to the treatment is mostly immediate. The sessions are often short and few in number. Only chronic disorders need spaced-out maintenance treatment at 6-8 weeks interval.

Su Jok acupuncture also serves as preventive medicine. Stimulating the corresponding pain points in the hands and feet by finger pressure, needles, or stimulators is an excellent way of preventing ill health.

Methods of Treatment

The Stick Massage. Once the painful point has been identified, a diagnostic* stick is used to apply pressure and stimulate the point. The diagnostic stick (any other similar shaped object may also be used provided it is not sharp: a matchstick, a ball pen, even a fingernail) must be pressed hard against the point. After the pain subsides under the stick, the point should be massaged continuously by rotating the stick clockwise and counterclockwise, while pressing against the point somewhat harder. The cure point must be completely massaged till the residual pain disappears and is replaced with a feeling of warmth.

At this stage, the treatment may be stopped because the symptoms of the acute illness will vanish. If several points of acute pain have been located in the correspondence area, each one must be treated, one by one, by this method.

A chronic disease would normally require more than one session. Correctly identified points need to be massaged with force for 3 to 5 minutes every 3 or 4 hours, till the condition improves. Repeated massage of the correspondence areas improves the condition, sometimes very rapidly.

The Seed Therapy. The seed therapy is another effective method of treatment. Pressure is applied on the points

---

* A pencil shaped stick made of stainless steel and about 10-12 cm. long.

of the hands and feet with the help of seeds of buckwheat (*kootu*), rice, wheat, apple, and so on. The same seeds are then plastered onto the points after a thorough massage. For a better effect it is recommended that they be kept in place for a day. The massage should be periodically repeated every three or four hours by pressing the seeds down with a rotary movement. The next day (after 24 hours) the seeds should be replaced with new ones and the procedure repeated.

This method is especially effective for chronic diseases accompanied by constant pains, for diseases of the joints, as well as for children who are more responsive to this therapy.

Seeds can either be placed singly over each painful point, or can cover the entire area corresponding to the afflicted organ.

Common Disorders Treated with *Su Jok*

Alcohol and heroin addictions	Gynaecological disorders
Cardiovascular disorders	Headaches
Constipation	Hepatitis
Cramps	Lumbago
Diarrhoea	Nausea
Ear, nose, and throat disorders	Nervous system and psychiatric disorders
Epilepsy	Obesity
Eye problems	Smoking
Fibrositis	Pain of all kinds in cancer
Genito-urinary disorders	Rheumatism
	Sexual disorders
	Skin disorders

The Elastic Ring Massage. Since the entire human body has corresponding points on the hands and feet and on each finger and toe, massaging of the fingers, toes, hands, and feet with an elastic ring is an effective way of preventing and treating diseases.

The ring is placed on a finger and the area corresponding to the afflicted part of the body is massaged till it grows red and warm. This procedure is to be repeated several times a day.

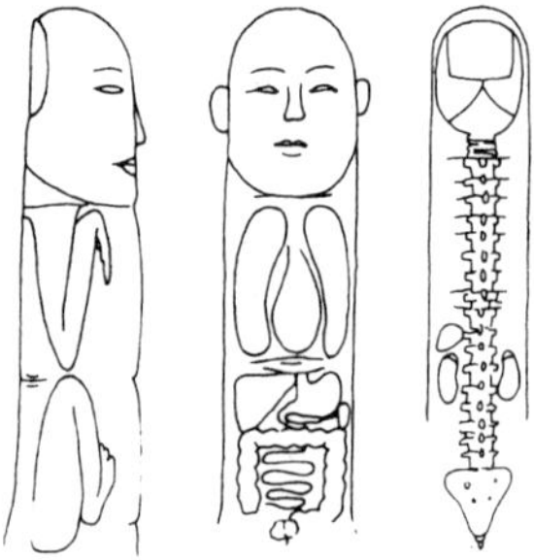

Fig. 24. Human Body as Represented on a Finger

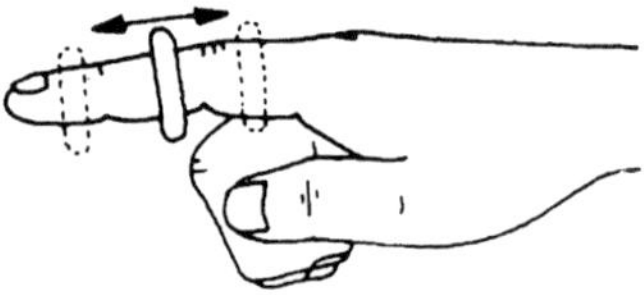

Fig. 25. Elastic Ring Massage

Su Jok acupuncture is a complete system of medicine with a range of applications just as wide as that of Western medicine. A doctor who combines Western scientific medicine with acupuncture can therefore select the most appropriate treatment in any particular case. He is able to treat a wide variety of diseases pertaining to any part or system of the body, including many psychological conditions in the best way possible.

11

Related Healing Systems

There are some other therapies related to acupuncture. The relationship or commonality of these therapies is that they also recognize and use the body's energies to effect cures by manipulation of the acupuncture points.

Acupressure: Massaging Acupuncture Points

Acupressure* is essentially a massage of acupuncture points. The science of acupressure developed after it was seen that effects similar to that of acupuncture could be obtained by pressing acupuncture points. The principle of massage has been used to alleviate pain for thousands of years.

The classical method of acupressure therapy is to use

---

* For more information consult *Acupressure Cure for Common Diseases* by Dr Keith Kenyon, published by Orient paperbacks, Delhi

a blunt needle to apply pressure over an acupuncture point. However, acupressure can also be done by using thumb or nail pressure. The pressure has to be applied and released repeatedly. The duration of pressure depends on the intensity of pain. If the point is very painful, it is pressed every few minutes for a few seconds. This process is repeated till the patient finds that the point is no longer as painful, and he can withstand greater pressure for a longer time. If there is no pain at an acupuncture point, pressure is applied for 30-60 seconds to obtain the required result. Traditionally, a deep centrifugal movement (moving away from the centre) is said to disperse or sedate, while a light centripetal movement is said to move towards the centre and has a tonification effect.

Pressure massage is ideally done with the thumb but may also be carried out by using the palm, base of the hand, elbow, knuckles, or fist. The finger should remain at the same point where the massage is performed with a circular motion or to and fro along the channel. Massage along the channel in the direction of the energy flow is especially effective when the pain is felt along the channel. Pressure exerted by fingers should be applied lightly over nerves around sensory organs and the frontal side of the neck.

Acupressure can also be used in addition to, and to compliment, acupuncture treatment. The major indications for acupressure therapy are painful conditions like headache, toothache, cervical spondylitis, and shoulder and lumbar pain. Many psychosomatic disturbances like sleep disturbances, nervousness, nausea, feeling of vomiting, seasickness, constipation, and menstrual problems can also be positively influenced by acupressure.

The basic advantage of this treatment is that it can

be carried out without any special equipment. The limitation is that only one point can be treated with acupressure at a time, whereas in patients with chronic problems, many points require to be treated simultaneously. Hence it is time-consuming. Moreover, acupressure is most effective when an acupuncture point lies over a bone and can be massaged against it. It is not so effective over soft areas like the abdomen.

In general, acupressure is not as effective a form of treatment as acupuncture because the force which is applied at a point is dissipated over a wider area. In acupuncture, the needle enters a point which is less than 2 mm in diameter. With the advent of sophisticated and painless means of therapy like lasers and ultrasound, the role of acupressure in therapy is diminishing.

Shiatsu

In the West, *shiatsu* is one of the most commonly used massage therapies. It developed in Japan in the early part of the 20th century. In Japanese the word *shi* means 'finger' and *atsu* means 'pressure'. *Shiatsu,* also sometimes called *shiatsu* acupressure, is an oriental massage in which the fingers are pressed on particular points of the body, called *tsubo.* These 361 *tsubos,* also called acupuncture points and pressure points, are located at specific places in the body's skin and muscular system along the 14 meridian lines or channels where nerves hurt or feel uncomfortable when the flow of energy (*Qi*) through the body is blocked. In actual practice only about ninety-two *tsubos* are used.

Like acupuncture, when skillfully performed, *shiatsu* can relieve pain and tension — complaints as varied as arthritis, headaches, haemorrhoids, menstrual cramps, impotence, and frigidity have all been treated successfully with it. The *shiatsu* practitioner is expected to have a thorough knowledge of the acupuncture points and meridians and the nuances of pulse and tongue diagnosis. In *shiatsu*, however, it is the abdominal diagnosis which is important in treatment of all diseases.

Reflexology

Reflexology is a form of acupressure which is applied on the palms of the hands and the soles of the feet. All parts of our body are symmetrically represented in the palms and soles. These reflex areas become correspondingly sensitive with a disorder in the part of the body to which they are related. Organs or parts on the right side of the body have their reflex areas on the right foot and hand.

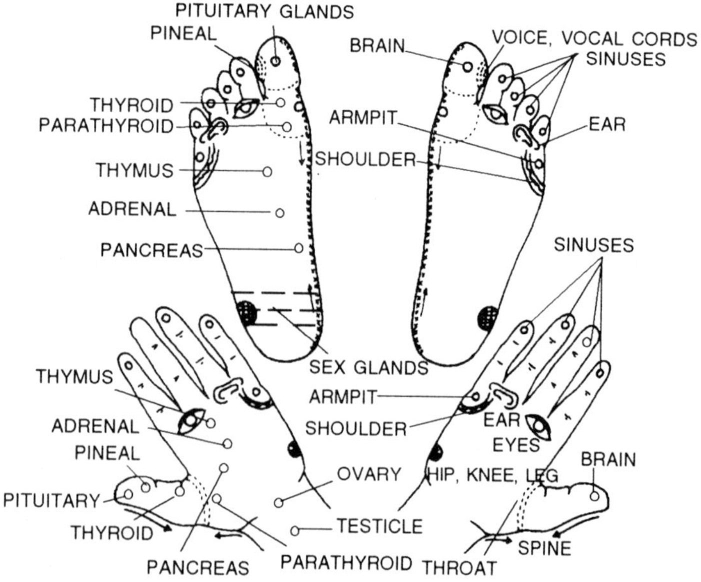

Fig. 26. The Palmar (Front) View of the Hands and Feet

Organs on the left side of the body have their reflex areas on the left foot and hand. Organs extending past the middle or centre of the body will have reflex areas on both feet and hands. Where there are two like organs or parts (kidneys, ovaries, etc.), each has a reflex area on its corresponding foot and hand. The lower half of the body has its reflex areas on the lower half of the foot, and the upper half of the body has its reflex areas on the upper half of the foot. The waistline is located approximately halfway between the base of the toes and the lower part of the heel. Reflex points are treated by massage, as is done by osteopaths and chiropractors, and this undoubtedly contributes to the favourable results experienced by these practitioners.

Chinese Osteopathy

Manipulation of joints is also a part of traditional massage employed in Chinese medicine and is sometimes called Chinese osteopathy. This probably has the effect of breaking down adhesions, restoring full mobility, stretching contracted tissue, and beneficially influencing the flow of energy or *Qi*.

Foot Massager Therapy

Foot reflexology is the basic principle of foot massager therapy. It is an advancement over foot reflexology in that the acupuncture points on the soles of the feet are stimulated with an automatic machine to attain instant effect and high efficiency.

For each acupuncture point on the sole, there is a corresponding massaging rod on the foot stimulator. By their unique continuous wave-like movements the massaging rods on the stimulator massage the respective acupuncture points individualy without missing any point, thus achieving a thorough massaging effect. Persistent massaging of the sole with this machine on a daily basis for a duration of 5 to 15 minutes each time, helps in relieving various types of acute and chronic pains. The massage can be repeated 2 to 3 times a day for a period of 5 to 15 minutes, depending on the severity of the problem. This massage can also be used to treat pain in the back and thighs.

In addition, by massaging all the acupuncture points, the entire blood circulation is improved. The metabolism is enhanced, thus rendering comfort to the body and relieving it of fatigue. In case, while being massaged, a patient experiences unbearable acute pain at certain acupuncture points on the foot, it is an indication of abnormalities of the connected organs. Daily massaging of these painful acupuncture points makes the pain gradually subside and restore the organs back to health. After the foot massage, the patient is advised to drink a glass of water to discharge the wastes produced by the increase in the metabolism of the body.

Moxibustion: Chinese Herbal Therapy

The word moxibustion is the Latinised derivation of the Japanese word *Moegusa.* Moxa, the dried leaves of the medicinal herb *Artemisia vulgaris,* are used in different forms to activate specific points or to warm certain areas. The moxa are ignited and applied directly or indirectly to acupuncture points as a form of treatment.

The precise physiological response of the body to heat has been well-documented: the initial constriction of local blood vessels is dilated, thus bringing about an increase in the local blood supply. This relieves pain, removes toxins, and soothens the nerves.

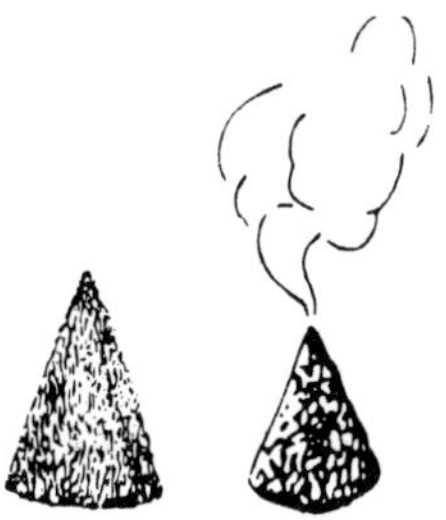

Fig. 27. Moxa Cones

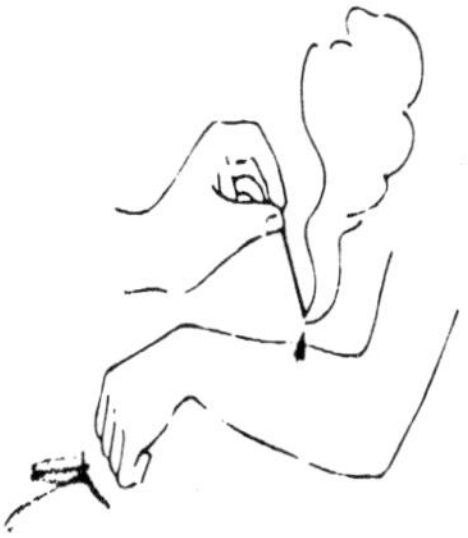

Fig. 28. Ignition of a Moxa Cone

Intensive research at the Shanghai College of Acupuncture, China has confirmed that moxa warms the vital energy and blood in the channels and expels the cold and dampness.

The following are the different ways in which moxibustion can be carried out:

Direct Moxibustion. The leaves of *Artemisia vulgaris* are first dried and prepared to give a similar consistency to that of cotton wool.

The moxa is then moulded into small cones about the size of rice grains, which are placed on the skin over the acupuncture points to be treated. Only one point is treated at a time. The moxa cone is ignited and allowed to burn. The moxa burns very slowly and the cone is flicked off the skin as soon as any discomfort is felt by the patient. This procedure is usually repeated with 3-5 cones per acupuncture point.

Indirect Moxibustion. There are four main methods of indirect moxibustion.

Indirect Moxibustion with Intermediate Substances. Fresh *ginger* slices, 1-2 mm thick, are used to isolate the direct heat of burning moxa leaves. Very small holes are

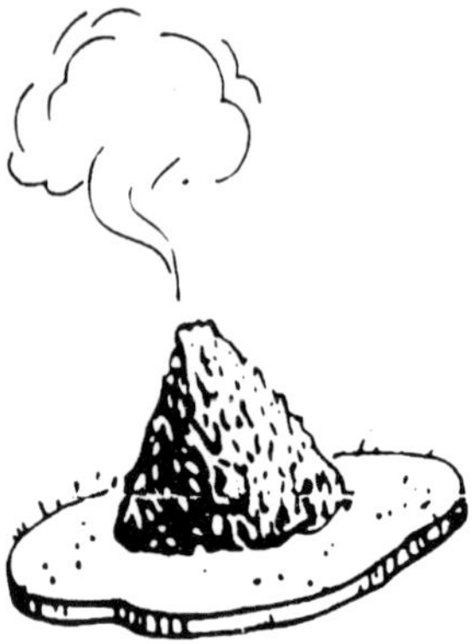

Fig. 29. Indirect Moxibustion with Ginger

pierced through the ginger slice and moxa placed on it. When the patient feels a sensation of heat at one point, the ginger slice with the moxa cone is moved away and placed on the next point, subsequently being returned to the first. In this way every point is heated 6-8 times, until a slight redness is observed. This method is very effective but it should be applied with care so as not to burn the skin.

Garlic may be used instead of ginger: it is particularly indicated in cases of chronic paralysis. The garlic piece should be about 1-2 mm thick and replaced after five cones of moxa have been burnt.

Clay can also be used as an intermediate substance and is recommended for eczema and some other skin problems. The treatment is generally continued till the patient feels an inner warmth.

Another intermediate substance used often is *white pepper*. The powdered form of white pepper is made into a paste with flour and water and spread over the point to be treated in a layer 2 mm thick. The moxa is placed on the paste and burnt. This method is good for arthritis and local numbness or stiffness.

Indirect moxibustion can also be done by using *salt* as the intermediate substance (see Fig. 30). This method is used on the navel which is filled with salt to the level of the surrounding abdomen, and then covered with a thin ginger slice. The moxa cone is placed on the ginger slice and ignited. This treatment is used for abdominal pain accompanied with diarrhoea, or for general augmentation of energy and vitality.

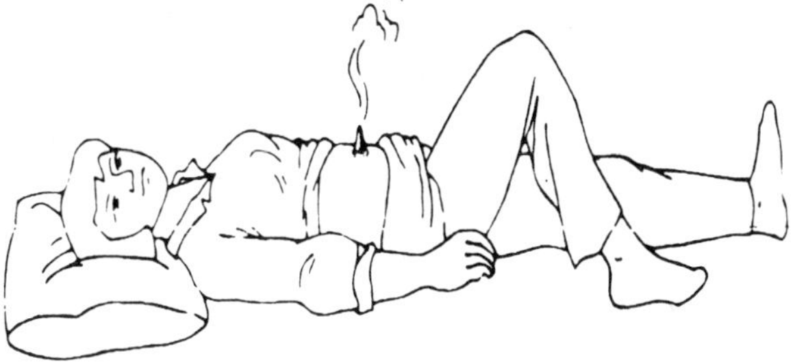

Fig. 30. Indirect Moxibustion with Salt

Indirect Moxibustion with a Moxa Stick. This is the simplest method of applying moxibustion and may be done over parts of the body where other methods are unsuitable, such as points which are covered by hair. The moxa roll or cigar-shaped stick is ignited at one end and brought to within 0.5-1 cm of the chosen acupuncture point until the patient feels a sensation of heat. The moxa roll is removed and brought closer after a few seconds again. This is repeated 6-8 times until a slight redness is observed. In this way every acupuncture point is heated for 30-40 seconds. Sparrow-pecking

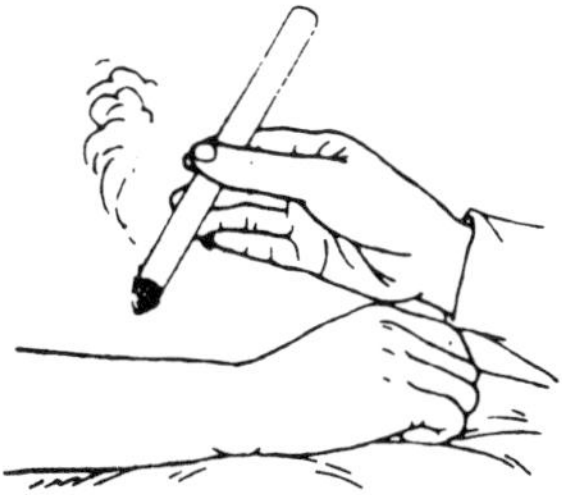

Fig. 31. Mild-warm Moxibustion

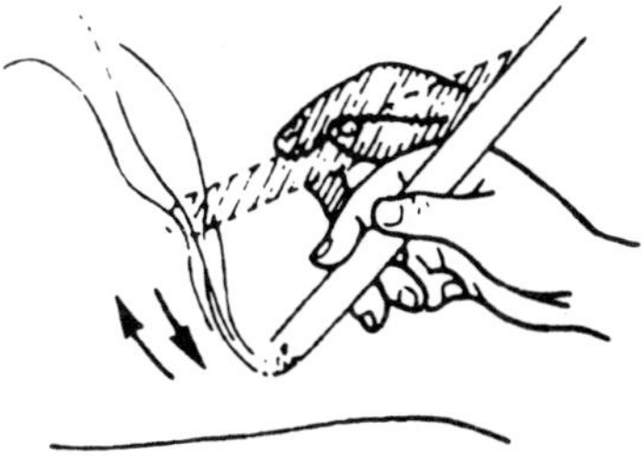

Fig. 32. Sparrow-pecking Moxibustion

moxibustion is another variation of indirect moxibustion with a moxa stick. This is applied much closer to the skin and may even touch the skin.

Indications for Moxibustion

Abdominal pain in normal menses
Aches and pain in the shoulders, back, waist, knees
All chronic diseases
Arthritic pain due to dampness in any joint
Bronchial asthma
Cervical spondylitis
Chronic bronchitis
Chronic diarrhoea
Depression
Dysmenorrhoea (painful menses)
Feeling of coldness in the body
Feeling of tiredness and exhaustion
Irritable bowel syndrome and other bowel diseases
Low backache
Myalgia
Pain in the hips, thighs, leg muscles, and feet
Periarthritis
Rheumatism
Rheumatoid arthritis
Sciatica
Soft-tissue injury pains
Warming hands, feet, and waist in winter

Indirect Moxibustion by Heating Acupuncture Needles. This is a common method of applying moxa and is done by fixing a small piece of moxa to the free end of an acupuncture needle and igniting it. This process can be repeated 2-3 times. This method is particularly useful in patients suffering from osteoarthritis. It is usual to surround the base of the needle at the level of the skin with a piece of thick paper to protect the skin from any accidental dropping of the burning moxa from the handle.

Indirect Moxibustion with Moxa Pain-Killing Belt: This is a unique and extremely effective self-applicable device which uses the principles of heat and moxibustion to get quick and effective relief from many chronic pains.

The moxa-belt therapy is based on the technology provided by the Shanghai College of Acupuncture, China, and is extremely effective because the heat from the moxa herb penetrates through the acupuncture points regularly, continuously, and in a balanced manner into the channels of the body. The moxa belt is extremely effective when applied to specific acupuncture points.

The medicinal moxa herb is packed into a small bag which can be fixed inside the heating belt. The heating unit is then switched on and the temperature control knob is rotated to a point where the patient feels most comfortable. It is used for a period of sixty minutes until relief is obtained.

Acupuncture and moxibustion are often practised together as complementary forms of treatment in the same session. The indications for moxibustion includes a wide range of weakness diseases given earlier. Contraindications for the use of moxibustion are: high fever, acute infectious diseases, hypertension, haemorrbages, menstruation, nervousness with sleep disturbances, and application on mentally disordered people. Moxibustion is not applied on the head, face, or near mucous membranes.

Cupping: The Vacuum Effect

A traditional method of treatment in the West and the East, cupping is a very valuable technique in which a vacuum area is created at acupuncture points, thereby enhancing the blood supply to that area. A hollow vessel, preferably a transparent glass cup, with a rounded, thick, and smooth rim, is used for the purpose. The doctor wraps a little cotton wool soaked in spirit around a pair of forceps. This is ignited and introduced for a second or two into the cup and withdrawn. The cup is then immediately applied to the patient over the area to be treated. The rapid cooling of the air inside the cup creates a partial vacuum and the flesh covered by the cup is raised into the cup. An alternative method is to ignite a small piece of wood infused with spirit on a protected area of the skin and invert the cup over it. The flame removes all the oxygen, thus creating a partial vacuum and producing a strong suction.

The cup is retained for 5-10 minutes, depending on the area being treated and the degree of suction induced. Cupping can also be combined with normal acupuncture, in which case the cup is simply placed over the inserted needle. Cupping is indicated in conditions of external dampness, and stagnation of *Qi* and phlegm. The main indications for cupping are arthritis, bronchial asthma, chronic back pain, chronic bronchitis, chronic diarrhoea, common cold, fibrositis, and sprains.

Cupping should not be used in cases of fever, convulsions, inflammation, infectious diseases, ulcers or abscesses, over hair, or in very nervous or pregnant patients.

12

Case Histories

Any alternative or complementary system of treatment is best authenticated by citing tried and tested examples of successful treatment. In keeping with this axiom, case histories* of disorders relating to the cardiovascular system; the muscles, bones, and joints; the nervous system; the respiratory system; psychiatric problems; the gastro-intestinal system; gynaecological problems; the skin; the eyes; and lifestyle are given in this chapter

Cardiovascular Disorders

Common cardiovascular disorders are angina pectoris, hypertension, and hypotension and palpitations.

Angina Pectoris. Angina pectoris is caused due to hardening and narrowing of the walls of the coronary

* The names have been changed to protect the privacy of the patients.

arteries; inflammation of the muscles of the heart; and syphilis. It usually occurs between forty to seventy years of age, and is more common in men. Although attacks of angina are often sudden and unexpected, usually the attack is preceded by feelings of pressure over the heart and general heart discomfort, perspiration over the entire body, and depression. When angina develops, the patient suddenly feels severe, almost unendurable pain in the heart under the sternum (the breastbone). There may be shortness of breath, cold arms and legs, and cold sweat.

O.P. Sachdeva, male, 67 years. This elderly man, came with complaints of frequent chest pain, more while standing, radiating to the left shoulder and the left arm, and relieved by taking rest and the tablet Sorbitrate. He had been suffering this for the past one year. ECG had confirmed that he was suffering from angina pectoris. His blood cholesterol levels were also high.

Acupuncture was started on him and in twenty sittings, he was completely relieved of his chest pain. Another course of twenty sittings was given to bring down his blood cholesterol level. A repeat blood test showed a normal lipid profile.

Hypertension. Hypertension can be defined as a consistent systolic blood pressure recording of over 140 mm of Hg in patients under fifty years of age, and a diastolic blood pressure recording of over 95 mm of Hg in patients above fifty years of age. Many patients with hypertension can be treated adequately with conventional medicine. However some are sensitive to the side-effects of drugs and in others drugs are unable to satisfactorily control the blood pressure.

There are two types of hypertension: primary and secondary. Primary or essential hypertension is the one for which no cause can be found. Such condition exists in ninety per cent of all patients with hypertension. It occurs mainly in patients over thirty years of age and the symptoms include headaches, dizziness, tinnitus, lack of sleep, and. numbness of limbs. Most of these patients have an imbalance in the ratio of the various neurotransmitters in the brain. Stimulation of different acupuncture points leads to the release of endorphins and encephalins. This constitutes the physiological basis of acupuncture in the treatment of hypertension.

Secondary hypertension is caused by nephritis (inflammation of the kidneys), toxaemia in pregnancy*, and endocrine disorders among other reasons, and is not treatable by acupuncture.

Subodh Mukherjee, male, 42 years. Subodh Mukherjee suffered from severe headaches and lack of sleep with extreme irritability for over six years before he contacted us. He had been diagnosed as hypertensive and put on Atenolol (50 mg), twice a day. In spite of the medication his blood pressure never stabilized and his symptoms persisted.

In fifteen sittings of acupuncture his headaches and sleep problems were cured. After three courses of twenty sittings each, the medicines were gradually tapered off and withdrawn. Blood pressure was maintained at 130/80 mm of Hg. Subsequently his blood pressure has been monitored periodically and he has not had any relapse.

* A condition in pregnancy characterized by increased blood pressure.

Bhupinder Singh, male, 68 years. A patient of chronic hypertension for fifteen years, Bhupinder Singh was on regular anti-hypertensive therapy when he first came for acupuncture treatment.

He was given regular acupuncture therapy for a month during which his blood pressure stabilized. His dosage of medicine was reduced from two tablets to one tablet a day, and acupuncture was given on alternate days for another month. After the second month, the medication was completely stopped and he was kept only on acupuncture therapy twice a week. During the fourth month sittings were given once a week. At the end of the fourth month his blood pressure had stabilized at 140/90 mm of Hg which was normal for his age. A follow-up with periodic recording of blood pressure has not shown any rise of blood pressure.

Hypotension and Palpitations. Hypotension is a condition in which a patient feels very low, does not feel like getting up from bed or doing any work, and complains of cold sweats, dizziness, and general fatigue. On examination, his blood pressure is always recorded as very low.

Palpitation of the heart is a common, subjective complaint described variously by the patient as 'pounding', 'fluttering', 'flopping', and 'skipping' of the heartbeat. The awareness of the heartbeat also tends to be more common at night and during introspective moments, but is less marked during activity. It is not unusual for palpitation to be the major manifestation of an emotional disorder. Other causes of palpitation include dyspepsia; mental or physical excitement; hyperthyroidism; anaemia; hysteria; trauma; circulatory disturbances; disorders of metabolism, nutrition, and growth; and heart diseases.

Vimla Aggarwal, female, 51 years. She had frequent complaints of dizziness, blackouts, palpitations, and bouts of profuse sweating. She had severe coldness of limbs which would not respond to any heat treatment. She felt weak, lethargic, and exhausted. Her blood pressure always remained around 90/60 mm of Hg.

She was given fifteen sittings of acupuncture in combination with moxibustion. She started feeling warmth in her limbs, more energetic, and her symptoms of dizziness, palpitations, and blackouts disappeared in ten further sittings. Her blood pressure rose up to 120/80 mm of Hg with a follow-up treatment regimen of alternate day for two weeks, twice a week for two weeks, and once a week for two weeks.

Vascular Disorders

The most common vascular disorders that can be successfully treated by acupuncture are early piles and varicose veins with ulcers.

Early Piles. Piles are due to an increased intra-abdominal pressure transmitted to the veins of the haemorrhoidal plexus causing bleeding. Straining while passing stools, prolonged sitting, obesity, and anal infections are the contributing factors. Bright blood from the rectum drips into the toilet bowl after the passage of stools with or without excruciating pain.

Rajender Kapoor, male, 42 years. Rajender Kapoor came with complaints of constipation, bleeding from the rectum, lethargy, and generalized weakness. He was a non-vegetarian and consumed alcohol daily.

On examination he was found to be suffering from first degree piles in which there is bleeding from the rectum but no mass protrudes out of the anus. He was advised an injection of sclerosing agent in piles by a surgeon. We gave him ten sittings of acupuncture and combined it with hot needle therapy (an acupuncture needle is heated and inserted for a second at the tip of tail of the backbone and taken out). His piles were cured. He was given another course of ten sittings to treat his constipation and was advised to change his dietary habits to prevent the recurrence of piles.

Varicose Veins with Ulcers. Varicose veins is a common problem in people who have to stand a lot. It is also common in ladies probably due to hormonal reasons. The veins become distended due to the weakness of the valves in their walls. These valves are responsible for the normal unidirectional flow of blood. Additionally the muscular tone of these veins is also reduced, causing them to become dilated. Patients suffering from this problem generally complain of inability to stand for a long period of time and of pain in the calf muscles. If the walls of these veins become very weak, they can rupture and cause varicose ulcers.

Dilbagh Singh, male, 33 years. Dilbagh Singh came to us in 1990, with a very severe problem of varicose veins accompanied with multiple varicose ulcers all over his right leg. The ulcers were infected and a purulent discharge kept oozing out. The various treatments he had tried had failed and antibiotics were unable to dry up the lesions. In fact he had been advised to have his leg, below the knee, amputated at the earliest. In this situation, we decided to take up the challenge.

We started giving him acupuncture therapy with needles placed on the affected leg. Additionally laser acupuncture was given to the wounds (varicose ulcers). Within the first fifteen sittings, the acute leg pain had subsided and the lesions started drying up. The patient was advised to continue the therapy and a total of forty-five sittings were given to him over a period of three months. The leg became totally normal and all the ulcers healed.

In our practice this has been our biggest single achievement so far. We were able to save a patient's leg from amputation. There has been no relapse of symptoms since then.

G.S. Maheswari, male, 45 years. For six years G.S. Maheswari had been suffering from varicose veins. He felt listless and tired and was not able to stand for more than five minutes at a stretch and felt like lying down. Acupuncture therapy was combined with sonopuncture in his case. A seven sq. cm ultrasound head was slowly massaged over the varicose veins.

It was very satisfying to see the veins starting to shrink. A total of sixty sittings were required to achieve a complete cure.

Diseases of Muscles, Bones, and Joints

Osteoarthritis, rheumatoid arthritis, cervical spondylosis, a stiff neck, low backache, a slipped disc, a frozen shoulder, and a calcaneal spur are the most common problems relating to the muscles, bones, and joints.

Osteoarthritis. This is a wear and tear disease affecting the cartilages of the joints and the underlying bone. It is estimated that twenty-five per cent of all women and fifteen per cent of all men above the age of sixty suffer from it noticeably, but the actual number affected may be far greater.

Osteoarthritis is localized to one or two joints and the patients feel fine apart from this particular joint trouble. It is often revealed through X-ray, since it can exist for years without any pronounced symptoms. In men it frequently attacks the shoulder or hip joint, and in women it seems to attack the knees more.

Postural faults may also bring about the disease, while injuries and falls are the other causes. The fact that women tend to put on weight round about menopause explains why they are more susceptible to osteoarthritis. Injuries such as dislocations, fractures, and war wounds seem to bring on osteoarthritic changes in later life.

The treatment should be aimed at relieving the cramp in the muscles associated with the joint. This will automatically improve the movement around the affected joint and increase the circulation of blood. Depending on the joint involved, the patient should also be advised a set of exercises which he should do regularly.

S.K. Mehta, male, 77 years. This elderly man came for treatment of pain in the right shoulder. The pain radiated across the right upper side of the back and down the right arm. He complained of tingling and numbness in the fingers. This problem had bothered him intermittently for the past 15-20 years. In addition, he had been suffering for the last three years from pain in the right buttock, which extended down the lateral side of his right leg to the knee. He was on Indocid (a drug used in cases of inflammation, rheumatoid arthritis, and pain) capsules, thrice a day, when he came to me for treatment. Examination showed him to be suffering from wasting of the leg muscles, with stiffness and pain in the right hip joint. He was diagnosed as having an obstruction in the circulation of energy and blood.

Moxa with needling was applied to a point on the hip and electro-acupuncture was given to points on the back. The leg and buttock pain (sciatica) responded immediately to the treatment. Needles were also used for the shoulder pain, which was cured completely.

A total of forty sittings were given in two courses of twenty sittings each and he was completely cured of his pain. In this case, moxibustion (heating of the acupuncture points) was used to remove the dampness, since this type of disorder is caused by dampness which obstructs the channels.

Mohit Sharma, male, 46 years. Another very interesting case which comes to my mind is that of Mohit Sharma, a stage actor, who came to us as a last resort in 1995. He was suffering from advanced arthritis of his right hip joint and despite treatment by a top orthopaedic specialist, his condition had deteriorated steadily. He was in continuous pain and had a pronounced limp. He was treated with needles and experienced immediate relief. He walked fairly free from pain after ten sittings and his nights were pain-free. After twenty sittings he asked us if something could be done for his limp.

We examined his left hip and buttock, that is, the healthy side, and to our surprise found trigger spots or painful points in the region of the buttock. He received the same treatment with needles on the unaffected side, and both the pain and the limp of the affected hip disappeared. He was completely cured within two months, having taken a total of thirty sittings. Subsequently, it was a pleasure to see him perform on stage, unhindered by any pain.

Bharat Suri, male, 45 years. Another interesting case history is that of Bharat Suri, who came to us in 1993 with the complaint that his right knee joint would suddenly lock, giving excruciating pain and preventing him from walking any further. An X-ray of the knee joint revealed a small chip of bone floating in the joint space — this was causing him the pain. He had had a road accident six months before the pain had started and not obtained any relief from any treatment. He had been advised surgery for removal of the broken chip of bone. He came to us with his problem and we gave him acupuncture daily for ten days. The locking vanished. The pain was relieved by about eighty per cent in twenty sittings and he was totally cured of his pain in thirty sittings. He never complained of any recurrence of pain even after four years.

Rheumatoid Arthritis. The term rheumatoid arthritis refers to a chronic, progressive disease causing inflammation and stiffening of the joints, including severe pain. Muscles may become wasted as the blood circulation is impaired. Tendon lesions are present in half the cases of rheumatoid arthritis, the long tendons of the fingers and those around the ankle joint being most often affected.

The first joints usually involved are the middle joints of the fingers of both hands, and gradually all the joints of the body get involved. The skin becomes dry and scaly. The hands are usually cold and clammy.

In initial stage the disease is completely reversible, and all symptoms disappear. If the next stage supervenes, the joint cartilage wears away and bony changes are seen in the X-ray. Later, the two halves of the joint may fuse or become ankylosed, producing a permanent stiffness.

Rheumatoid arthritis is more common in middle and

young age although, sometimes, children may also develop this disease.

Brij Mohan, male, 38 years. Suffering from rheumatoid arthritis for over four years, Brij Mohan used to complain of pain in the neck, wrist, elbow, shoulders, fingers, knee, and ankle joints. Regular acupuncture therapy was given to him for twenty days and his pain and stiffness were relieved dramatically. His ESR also reduced considerably. After three courses of twenty sittings each, the pain was fully cured. A follow-up showed no relapse of pain even after three years.

Cervical Spondylitis. For this problem acupuncture is considered most successful. Generally the patient suffers from pain in the region of the neck, along with stiffness and limitation of movement. The pain may radiate to the head, causing headaches, dizziness, pain in the arm, and pain in the chest.

Treatment with prolonged drug therapy is unsatisfactory as the relief obtained is only symptomatic. A large number of patients suffering from this problem, ranging in chronicity from one year to as old as twenty years, have been treated with acupuncture with excellent results.

It is our recommendation that acupuncture should be the first line of treatment in this disorder and not the last resort. By using it at an early stage, it is possible to prevent the many crippling deformities that are seen in this disease. Acupuncture is the method par excellence for relieving pain without causing any side-effects.

Kamal Pandit, male, 45 years. He came to us in 1994 with complaints of acute pain in the neck accompanied by severe headaches and pain in both the shoulder blades. He had been suffering for the past two years. The X-ray of his cervical spine revealed evidence of spondylosis. He had been prescribed painkillers, physiotherapy exercises, and cervical traction, but with little or no relief. He was using a cervical collar to avoid jerks to his neck.

Acupuncture therapy was started and after the third sitting, the neck stiffness disappeared. The pain in his neck and his headache were considerably reduced. He was given twenty sittings, after which he felt eighty per cent better. After a break of seven days, the frequency of therapy was reduced and a total of ten more sittings were given over the next four weeks. He has been totally asymptomatic after that and has been advised simple neck exercises daily for ten minutes.

Leela Menezes, female, 30 years. This young lady used to suffer from constant headaches, neck pain, and numbness of both hands with pain radiating to both the arms. An MRI scan revealed degenerative changes in the cervical and lumbar* spine. The patient also complained of a feeling of weakness in the region of the neck.

Acupuncture therapy was started along with sonopuncture, and in just five sittings, the patient, who had been bedridden for the past twenty days, was able to rejoin work. Regular therapy was continued for twenty sittings. Her headaches stopped; the neck felt normal; there was no pain in the shoulder blades and arms; and the numbness of hands totally disappeared.

Shyam Mehta, male, 43 years. A not-so-common presentation of cervical spondylosis is when patients complain of severe vertigo, that is, a feeling of acute

* Relating to the loin, especially the lower back area.

dizziness, nausea, and vomiting, with no history of neck pain. All other investigations show normal results except the X-ray of the cervical spine which is likely to reveal narrowing of the disc spaces with varying degrees of disc degeneration. This is caused by blockage of the blood supply from the neck to the occipital region (the back of the head). Due to the lack of blood going up, the patient gets attacks of acute dizziness.

Shyam Mehta came to us in 1996 with complaints of acute dizziness and giddiness. He was advised to take Stemetil tablets, twice a day, to get symptomatic relief. However, he started feeling quite depressed because he would suddenly develop a feeling of unsteadiness and experience extreme nausea. The symptoms were aggravated on lying down. The X-ray confirmed the diagnosis of cervical spondylitis. Acupuncture points were selected for treating the basic cause of the symptoms along with certain symptomatic points. Within the first five sittings, the feeling of vertigo started getting less and the patient felt more confident. A regular course of twenty sittings was given and the patient recovered fully. A follow-up with the patient has revealed no recurrence of symptoms for the past two years.

Acute Stiff Neck. An acute stiff neck is generally caused by a contraction or spasm of one or more muscles of the neck due to local injury, a sprain, or unsuitable posture of the head during sleep. Characteristically the patient cannot move the head on getting up in the morning. There is an acute unbearable pain in the neck, radiating to the shoulder or back.

Mahak Singh, male, 9 years. A typical example of an acute stiff neck leading to acute headaches and blurring of vision, with pain in the shoulder blades, is of this young boy. His parents had consulted many specialists but the symptoms persisted for over one year. Then they came to us. As the boy was very apprehensive of needles, he was treated with infra-red laser at certain acupuncture points. In just twenty sittings, the boy's headaches vanished, and he and his parents went away smiling.

Anju Jain, female, 32 years. A lecturer in a college, Anju Jain, came to me with an acute stiff neck which she had developed overnight due to contraction of the sternomastoid muscle in a faulty sleeping posture. This had caused a rotation of the head to the opposite side and flexion of the neck to the same side.

Specific acupuncture points for an acute stiff neck were selected and the patient was made to move her neck while the needle was being rotated manually at a specific acupuncture point. In just 2-3 minutes, the stiffness disappeared and after a sitting of thirty minutes, she left the clinic smiling as all her pain had gone.

Low Backaches. Low back pain is a common painful disorder and it is estimated that at least ninety per cent of people suffer from backaches at least once in their lifetime.

The conventional treatment of backache consisting of analgesics is unsatisfactory as it does not attempt to treat a variety of symptoms ranging from a localized pain in the low back and sciatica to pain in the hips, thighs, knees, calves, and ankles. A proper diagnosis is necessary and investigations include an ESR check and an X-ray of the spine.

The factors which could lead to a backache range from injury, infection, and degeneration of the spinal column to pregnancy and calcium deficiency. Other common causes include lifting of heavy objects, motor-car accidents, a fall from a height or down a flight of stairs, or anything that gives a jerk to the body. An exaggerated stoop or excessively leaning forward is also harmful. People who suffer from chronic constipation as well as women who have menstrual disorders, are also prone to problems of the back.

Acupuncture is extremely effective in the treatment of low back pain. Our own experience of using it is largely for chronic pains, but we have used it very successfully in acute backache cases, who were even unable to turn in bed and groaned in pain. The patient is made to lie down in a prone position and then examined for tender points. Tender points are generally those spots where the patient says 'ouch' on applying pressure. Once these points have been located, the acupuncturist needles these points with very fine and thin acupuncture needles. These needles are vibrated with a battery-operated stimulator for a period of 20-30 minutes, after which they are removed. Needling releases pain-killing endorphins in the blood and these cure the pain.

A course of 15-20 sittings of acupuncture is given regularly, in which most patients recover completely or achieve about seventy per cent recovery. The frequency of therapy is then gradually reduced till the pain gets fully cured. During the intervening period, a small ring is fixed at the backache point located in the ear, as all diseases can be treated by treating acupuncture points in the ear. After the patient is fully cured, a set of exercises is advised to strengthen the spine.

S.K. Bhattacharya, male, 50 years. He telephoned us that he had suddenly developed an acute backache after lifting a bucket of water. The pain was so sharp and severe that he was unable to turn in bed. He had been given pain-killing injections but to no avail.

On examination, we found tender points along the lumbar spine and in the buttock area. These points were needled for thirty minutes. On removal of the needles, the same points were cupped. After one sitting, he was able to turn on his side and sit up in bed. After three sittings, he was able to rejoin work.

Earlier he had suffered from episodes of acute low back pain every six months or so and needed bedrest for about three weeks every time before he could return to work. After treatment, his pain has not recurred.

Roop Rani, female, 80 years. This old lady came to us for treatment with complaints of pain in the lower back and radiating to the hips and thighs. She had been suffering for two years. An X-ray of the lumbar spine showed degenerative changes. She also had tender points over both the hip joints. Needling over the hip joint helped to dramatically reduce the pain and in just 15 sittings, she was cured.

Slipped Disc with Sciatica. The spine supports our body, provides a framework for the attachment of our organs and muscles, and provides the nerve supply to all parts of the human body. Any disorder affecting the spine may cause a problem in any other part of the body which receives its nerve supply from the affected spinal segment. There are thirty-two vertebrae in our spinal column with an intervertebral disc in-between them to absorb the impact of one's movements. These discs are basically soft elastic cushions. When the intervertebral discs are thrown out of alignment, one suffers from what is known as a Slipped Disc. Sometimes both the discs and the vertebrae are thrown out of alignment, causing a wide range of problems like headaches, shoulder or arm pain, a tingling and numbness in the fingers, and pain in the low back, chest, and abdomen. This may cause sciatica pain (indicating symptoms of nerve root compression in the leg, with the pain shifting to the buttocks, thighs, calves, and ankles).

The basic cause of this pain is the spasm of the muscles in the back. This spasm prevents any further movement of the part that is out of alignment. Although back sprain, fibrositis, or fibromyalgia are the commonest causes of low back pain, it is possible that the more serious and intractable forms are due to chemical inflammation of the nerve structures by an irritating glycoprotein from a damaged disc.

Smita Sharma, female, 40 years. A history of a slipped disc for three years had put the lady into hospital for varying periods. When she consulted us she was in acute pain and also complained of difficulty in bending. Her left foot was numb. Tender spots were found in the left buttock and in the calf muscles on examination. The back muscles over the affected disc were in a state of spasm. She was given six acupuncture sittings and advised back exercises. She made good progress and became free from all symptoms in three weeks.

Subhash Paswan, male, 40 years. A resident of Meerut, Subhash Paswan, consulted us for an acute pain in his left leg which radiated from the back to the hip, the outer side of the thigh, the leg, and ended at the ankle. He also complained of severe tingling in the toes of the feet. The CAT scan of the lumbosacral spine revealed a prolapsed disc with protrusion of the disc. No painkiller or traction had given him any relief for the past six months. As a last resort he was advised surgery by a renowned orthopaedic surgeon.

We treated him with acupuncture and he required two courses of twenty sittings each for a complete cure. He has had no relapse of the pain for the past two years.

S.B. Midha, male, 58 years. Suffering from a prolapsed disc for six years, he had been admitted to the Army Hospital at least a dozen times to obtain relief from pain by pain-killing injections and traction. Before coming to us he was given a date to remove the herniated disc by surgery. Fortunately one of his relatives who had been cured of back pain with acupuncture suggested him to consult us. Examination revealed an acute spasm of the piriformis (pear-shaped) muscle, along with acute tenderness along the entire course of the sciatic nerve.

Acupuncture therapy was started immediately and in a period of two months, he was fully cured of his problem. When we met him later, he said that the pain had never recurred.

Frozen Shoulder. A painful shoulder often occurs as a symptom due to sprain or strain of the soft tissues surrounding the shoulder joint, which may cause inflammation of the shoulder joint in a specific area.

This periarthritis* of the shoulder joints is due to chronic degeneration and inflammation of the bursa and surrounding soft tissues of the shoulder joint. It may have started with a slight sprain or local chilling or even have occurred spontaneously. The pain may cover a large area and radiate to the neck and arm, being accompanied

* Inflammation of tissues around a joint.

by local tenderness. There is a limitation of movement when raising, abducting (drawing away from the middle line of the body), or stretching the arm posteriorly. Another notable feature of this disease is that pain is the main complaint in the early stages, while in the later stages, the chief problem is the functional disturbance of movements.

Acupuncture treatment is very effective in early stages of periarthritis for relieving the pain, but at the later stages of the disease when adhesive inflammation between the joint capsule and articular cartilage occurs, the joints become stiff, exercises, in addition to acupuncture treatment, are necessary to restore normal movement.

Karuna Shanker, male, 50 years. Suffering from a frozen shoulder for one year, he came to us for treatment. Due to the pain in his left shoulder joint, he could not lift his left shoulder. As a result he could not perform his magic shows. He had tried all modes of therapy like infra-red rays, physiotherapy, and allopathic painkillers, but with little or no relief.

Acupuncture treatment was given to him along with cupping therapy at the painful points. His pain started getting less from the first sitting itself and after one month of treatment, he was able to perform his shows again and lift his shoulder completely without any pain.

Tennis Elbow. Pain at the elbow joint is commonly seen among tennis players. That is why this condition is commonly called tennis elbow. Those who do not play tennis may also suffer from elbow pain. Getting a tennis elbow is frequent between the ages of forty to sixty years, the years when cervical spondylosis is also common.

Narsingh, male, 45 years. He is a coach with the Delhi Lawn Tennis Association. He could not play tennis for about six months due to severe pain in his right elbow. Doctors had even given him steroids injections in his right elbow joint but there was no improvement in his condition. Since he was coaching our children, they brought him to us. Twenty sittings of acupuncture along with cupping therapy relieved his pain completely and he was back to tennis.

Gout. Gout is due to deposition of monosodium urate crystals in and about the joints and tendons, and in the interstitial tissue of the renal parenchyma. An inflammatory reaction to the crystal deposits accounts for the acute attacks. Acute onset, usually monoarticular, involves the metatarsophalangeal joint of the big toe (in about fifty per cent of the cases). Urate is deposited in subcutaneous tissues, bones, cartilages, joints, and other tissues. The pain, often of nocturnal onset, is many times described as throbbing, crushing, or excruciating. The skin is hot, tense, shiny, and dusky red or purple in colour. The first few attacks usually last only for a few days, but later untreated attacks may persist for several weeks.

Vinod Chibber, male, 50 years. He was suffering from gout for the past two years. His pain started with right big toe and gradually involved both his knees. There was a lot of swelling on these joints. He could not even wear his shoes and walk without support. His uric acid level in the blood was also high (10 mg%). He was taking the tablet Zyloric, but with little relief.

Acupuncture was given for twenty days daily initially during which the swelling subsided completely and his uric acid level came down to 5 mg%. Follow-up treatment was given on alternate days for two weeks, followed by twice a week, and then once a week. He was completely cured of his pain.

Calcaneal Spur (Pain in the Heel). Pain in the surface of the foot (sole) comprises pain in the sole and pain in the heel. Pain in the sole is caused by an injury to the planter arch. There is a burning pain beneath the metatarsal bones, often radiating to the dorsum (back) of the foot.

Pain in the heel is caused by an acute bursitis or due to an overgrowth of the calcaneus (calcaneal spur) which irritates the nerves and causes pain. This pain is aggravated by standing or walking.

Anjana Tripathi, female, 29 years. This young lady came to us with complaints of excruciating pain in her right heel with swelling around the ankle joint. She had injured her ankle due to a jerk about three months ago. Local anti-inflammatory creams, infra-red, short-wave diathermy, and painkillers had not provided any relief. Finally she was given a steroid injection at the site of the pain, but the pain recurred after one week.

She was in agonizing pain and not even able to keep her right heel down on the floor. Acupuncture therapy was given to her for a period of forty-five minutes. After the needles were removed the pain had reduced by 20-25 per cent. Sonopuncture treatment at the painful spots on the heel and the sole of foot followed. Within fifteen minutes of this therapy, she was able to keep her foot down on the floor and walk a few steps with mild discomfort. Regular treatment was given to her for fifteen days and the pain totally disappeared.

Diseases of the Nervous System

Migraines, epilepsy, trigeminal neuralgia, paralysis in children, and hemiplegia are some of the common disorders of the nervous system that can be treated with acupuncture. Coma is another condition for which acupuncture treatment has proved successful.

Migraines and Common Headaches. Headache is probably the commonest complaint in medical practice. Many patients with a recurrent headache are labelled as having a migraine. In most cases, clinical examination reveals a problem affecting the sinuses or the cervical spine.

The causes of headaches are varied. Reading too much, catching a cold, or neuralgia of the head are among the commonest causes. Neuralgic headaches may be chronic, occurring daily for many years. They are untreatable with Western medicine.

There are tension headaches and migraines (the two most common categories), cluster headaches, neuralgic headaches, and headaches associated with eye strain, hormonal changes, menopause, birth control pills, allergies, sinus, and even sex.

Migraine headache is a paroxysmal* disorder which is characterized by recurrent attacks of headache with or without associated visual disturbances. Often, a migraine is preceded by psychological disturbances. It is more common in women and tends to occur during the period immediately preceding their menstrual cycle. It has a maximum prevalence in the third and fourth decades of human life and gradually tends to wear off as the patient grows older. It is postulated to be due to or aggravated by hormonal changes.

---

* A fit of disease.

Both laser and acupuncture treatment can cure migraine headaches. If headaches occur again, the treatment needs to be repeated for a short course.

M.P. Randhawa, male, 62 years. Suffering from migraines for twenty-five years, he did not get relief from any medicine and the episodes of headaches occurred every third day and lasted for a day or two. He was treated with acupuncture for two months. His pain vanished and he has not required any medicine since then.

Pratibha Sahni, female, 34 years. She had recurrent migraine headaches associated with dizziness, vomiting, and vertigo for six years. From the first acupuncture sitting itself, the intensity of pain steadily diminished. In fact the headache vanished by the second sitting. But a full course treatment of twenty sittings was given and the patient is now symptom free.

Preeti Sood, female, 19 years. Preeti used to suffer from severe bouts of vomiting, blurring of vision, giddiness, and unilateral headaches which were localized at a particular point on the side of the head. She had suffered from this problem for over three years and expensive investigations like the CAT Scan and MRI had revealed nothing abnormal.

On examination, painful spots could be located in the neck and forehead. She was also a very sensitive person by nature and attacks were often precipitated by stress and anxiety. Acupuncture was combined with psychotherapy and she was cured of her migraine headaches in only two months.

Epilepsy. In this disease the patient usually has a history of recurrent attacks or seizures. The attacks appear suddenly.

In grand mal epilepsy, the patient loses consciousness after a sharp scream and falls down; the body muscles become rigid; there is dilatation of the pupils; intermittent convulsions of all the four extremities; facial cyanosis; incontinence of urine and stool; and biting of the tip of the tongue. The seizure may last for a few minutes, after which the patient falls into a deep sleep and has no recollection of the attack on awakening.

In petit mal epilepsy, the seizure lasts only for a few seconds. There is a loss of consciousness but no convulsions. The patient may suddenly stare straight ahead into space, and objects held in the hands may drop. Acupuncture is an extremely effective cure for this disease.

Jaideep Ghose, male, 14 years. Jaideep Ghose was afflicted with epilepsy since he was five months old. He had been on drugs which included Eptoin, Luminal, and Mazetol, but the fits continued to occur. Twitching of the muscles, frothing from the mouth, unconscious spells after a fit, a feeling of lethargy — all these were manifestations of the grand mal epilepsy which this child suffered from. He could not attend school regularly because the allopathic drugs prescribed made him drowsy and he could not concentrate at all on his studies.

An acupuncture regimen was started and he was given regular treatment for four weeks, along with the medication. After one month of the treatment the dose was reduced to half. By the third month, the medication was completely withdrawn. When no fits occurred in the following period, the daily acupuncture regimen was reduced to an alternate-day therapy for two weeks, and gradually the sittings were tapered off to one sitting per month. This once-a-month treatment continued for two years without a single fit and Jaideep was declared cured. In perfect health now, Jaideep has a joyous future mapped out for him.

Parkinson's Disease. This is a disease with symptoms of 'Pill-rolling' tremors involving the thumb, index finger, or wrist. In a full-blown disease, the facial expression is fixed; the eyes are unblinking and staring; the mouth is slightly open and often drolling; the facial skin is greasy. Other symptoms include gait and postural abnormalities, rigidity, and speech difficulties. The insidious onset usually begins in the fifty to sixty age bracket, with slow progression.

Pyare Lal, male, 48 years. Pyare Lal came to us with a history of trembling in both hands and inability to walk freely. He had severe stiffness all over the body and his movements were very slow. He had been diagnosed as a case of Parkinsonism about six months earlier and put on allopathic medication.

Acupuncture treatment was given to him daily for two courses of twenty sittings each. After the first course his trembling reduced by fifty per cent and his movements became more free and coordinated. The dosage of allopathic medicines was reduced to half. After the second course, he was able to walk freely and his stiffness reduced to a great extent. With a follow-up treatment of twice a week for four months, he was cured completely and advised to leave all medicines.

Insomnia. Insomnia is a problem which is seen very often in today's stressful society. Patients suffering from this problem are sometimes on sleeping pills forever.

Lucilda Cooper, female, 45 years. Lucilda Cooper had

been suffering from insomnia for over five years and was regularly taking Alprax at bedtime but even with medication, she could not sleep soundly.

Acupuncture therapy was given and within just ten sittings her tranquillizers were stopped and she was able to get a sound sleep. Since then she has not had any recurrence of this problem.

Paralysis in Children. Infantile paralysis is an acute infectious disease of the central nervous system. It is caused by invasion of the polio virus into the anterior horn cells of the spinal cord via the digestive tract. Tell-tale symptoms are fever, general malaise, and various signs referable to the respiratory and digestive tracts which subside in 1-4 days. Fever recurs after 3-6 days and is accompanied by headache, drowsiness, and vomiting. This is the pre-paralytic stage. In the paralytic stage the fever subsides after a week and flaccid paralysis of the muscles and limbs sets in. In most cases, the lower limbs are affected, on one or both sides. Reflexes are lost on the affected side without any sensory loss. Recovery starts after 1-2 weeks. Some children may recover fully in one year, while others develop muscular atrophy and deformity.

Rohini, female, 5 years. Polio is also a condition in which there is a viral infection leading to infantile paralysis. Rohini developed polio with a foot drop (foot remains in a forward drooping position) involving both the lower limbs. She was brought to us after she had not responded well to physiotherapy. She was brought by her parents carried in their lap as she was not even able to sit or stand without support. The child was very co-operative and allowed us to insert 5-6 needles in every sitting on both the legs. In just fifteen sittings she was able to sit on her own and stand with support. In twenty sittings she was able to stand without support, and in a month she was able to walk, though with a limp.

It took us another two months to cure her foot drop and her limp. This child was one of our earliest patients. She is now a grown-up girl and none can make out if she ever had paralysis on both her lower limbs.

Hemiplegia. Hemiplegia means paralysis of one half of the body. Paralysis occurs on the side opposite to the affected side or hemisphere of the brain. The cause of hemiplegia is a pathological clot in a blood vessel. In most cases, the onset is abrupt and the evolution, rapid. The three major causes of hemiplegia are thrombosis, embolism, and haemorrhage. Other causes include trauma to the brain stem, a brain tumour, brain abscess, encephalitis, and complications of meningitis.

Treatment of the acute stage starts with bedrest, airway maintenance, adequate oxygenation, naso-gastric feeding or IV fluids, attention to bladder and bowel functions, and measures to prevent bed sores. Heart failure, severe hypertension, and intercurrent respiratory infection are also treated.

After the initial improvement, the patient's progress is very slow. Rehabilitation and aftercare is designed by the physician and the physiotherapist.

Karan Singh, male, 42 years. Karan Singh, was a known hypertension patient who used to take medicines very irregularly. One day his blood pressure shot up very high and he suffered a cerebral haemorrhage, which caused paralysis on the right side of his face, right arm, and right leg. His speech was affected and became slurred.

He was kept in the hospital for two days, and then discharged and advised to continue physiotherapy at home. However, his relatives immediately brought him to us. On examination, we found that he could not even lift his right hand, and was not able to stand on his own. The right side of his face was paralysed and whatever he ate or drank would come out.

Acupuncture treatment was started immediately and, in just ten sittings, his facial paralysis was cured. He was able to lift his right shoulder slightly and the right leg was now able to grip the floor. Regular therapy along with daily exercises were continued for a period of two months and the patient went home fully cured.

Sushma Khote, female, 50 years. Admitted to a nursing home after the left side of her body had been paralysed about eight months back, she was kept for one week and discharged. When she returned home, she was unable to stand on her own and was able to walk only with the help of a walker. Her CAT scan had revealed a cerebral infarct on the right side. Since one of the family members was already our patient, they had faith in the efficacy of acupuncture. We were called in immediately to start her treatment. Scalp acupuncture was combined with acupuncture on the left hand and the left leg. After just fifteen sittings, she was able to stand without support, lift her shoulder, and able to eat food with her left hand.

After another ten sittings, we made her discard the walker and walk a few steps without support. She was so happy that day that she literally wept. She was back on her own legs. Subsequently acupuncture treatment was continued for another month and the patient recovered fully. The muscle power in both her hand and leg became normal and she could do all routine chores without any difficulty.

Coma. Coma is defined as a condition where the patient goes into a state of unconsciousness. There can be various causes of coma.

Rajeev Jain, male, 75 years. He had sustained a head injury in an accident. He was operated upon and the clot in his brain removed but he still did not come out of coma. He was given acupuncture continuously for three hours on the first day and came out of deep coma on the same day itself. Thereafter, he was given acupuncture treatment daily for the next fifteen days and he recovered fully.

Suneel Mishra, male, 40 years. He had been in deep coma for three and a half months following a brain haemorrhage and was on a ventilator and tube-feeding. He showed first signs of improvement after ten sittings of acupuncture treatment and was given a total of sixty sittings for recovery.

Atul Rawat, male, 35 years. He had pontine haemorrhages following severe uncontrolled hypertension and went into deep coma. He was admitted into a hospital and put on a ventilator. His relatives were told that there were no chances of his survival. Acupuncture was tried as a last resort and it worked wonders on him. He came out of deep coma by the 15th day, and the ventilator was removed. At the end of forty sittings, he recovered substantially enough to be discharged from the hospital. He was then under acupuncture treatment for residual paralysis and had regained even his normal mental abilities.

Respiratory Disorders

Acute laryngitis, bronchial asthma, and chronic sinusitis, are extremely common problems today and have a high success rate of cure with acupuncture.

Acute Laryngitis. Acute laryngitis is caused by inflammation of the larynx. This is most often caused either due to an infection or due to straining of the vocal cords.

Satish Babbar, male, 32 years. A very interesting case of acute laryngitis is that of Satish Babbar, the renowned ghazal singer. He was busy with the recording of a TV serial when he suddenly felt his voice getting choked and he became hardly audible.

An ENT specialist was consulted, who prescribed some antibiotics and a complete voice rest. However, as recording for the serial had been arranged, Satish Babbar got jittery and contacted us.

On examination, his larynx was found to be inflamed and he complained of acute pain in the throat with a dry cough and hoarseness of voice. One sitting of acupuncture treatment lasting for forty minutes was given and when the needles were removed, the patient was surprised that the pain had disappeared. His voice was better but not fully normal. Local irradiation of the vocal cords was done by using a infra-red laser and in just five minutes of laser therapy, his voice returned to normal. He was able to complete his recording the same day, and after three sittings, was fully cured.

Bronchial Asthma. The leading characteristic of this disease is its paroxysmal nature. An asthmatic may be well one minute, but may suffer from a violent attack half an hour later. The onset is often in early morning, with the patient feeling tightness in the chest, coughing, difficulty in breathing, and wheezing with inability to bring out sputum. In a severe attack, he may get out of bed, stand by an open window, and cling to surrounding objects to bring into play the accessory muscles of respiration. As the attack develops and breathing becomes difficult, the patient becomes alarmed. An attack may last for a few minutes, hours, or days. As the attack subsides, breathing becomes gradually easier; the patient often coughs out mucoid sputum, and then rapidly recovers.

Sometimes the lips, cheeks, and nail beds become increasingly blue, indicating cyanosis. The inspiratory effort is shortened, while the expiration is markedly prolonged. Crackling and gurgling sounds are heard. Between attacks, the chest is often normal. In uncomplicated asthma, the chest X-ray shows no special features.

In bronchial asthma, there is narrowing of the trachea, bronchi, and bronchioles. The causes of asthma are many. Persons whose asthma is precipitated by allergenic exposure (dust or pollen) have allergenic or extrinsic asthma. Thirty to fifty per cent of adult asthmatics have episodes that are triggered only by non-allergenic factors such as infection, irritants, and emotional factors, and have intrinsic asthma. Allergy is implicated more in infants and children than in adults. Climatic conditions also play a major part. Thus, one patient may have attacks in winter and another during the monsoons.

The disease is gradually progressive and its treatment in Western medicine is purely symptomatic. With each attack the requirement of bronchodilator drugs increases. Many patients are given corticosteroids, with all their attendant hazards.

Acupuncture treatment of bronchial asthma is prolonged

and can extend from six months to an year, depending upon the severity. The long-term results, however, are encouraging. Sixty per cent patients are cured and do not have any further problems. Twenty-five per cent have a recurrence during the first few months after treatment and require periodic follow-up treatment every 3-4 months. Ten to fifteen per cent patients benefit substantially as long as the treatment is going on, but once it is stopped and the drugs tapered off, they are likely to have a recurrence. Almost all patients can be symptom-free without medication.

Vipin Poddar, male, 29 years. This young man came to us with a history of recurrent attacks of bronchitis associated with wheezing every 2-3 months. The patient gave a family history of asthma (father) and stated that he too, had been suffering since childhood.

During the acute attack, the patient was treated by putting a needle in his neck, and within a few minutes, the attack subsided. Between attacks, the patient was needled on the back, upper limbs, chest, and lower limbs. The needles were stimulated with an electro-stimulator for twenty minutes once a day.

He was given a course of twenty sittings after which he felt seventy per cent better and stopped all his drugs. This drug withdrawal was done gradually and not suddenly. The patient was given a second course of alternate-day sittings for a period of four weeks. The vital energy or the *Qi* became activated with acupuncture, so that the immunity of the patient was increased and the allergy to different substances disappeared.

The frequency of therapy was reduced gradually to twice a week, and then once a week, and then stopped.

The patient is now totally asymptomatic and has had no attacks since.

Vinod, male, 13 years. This young boy was an interesting case because he met us purely by chance while we were treating someone else. He told us that he suffered from asthma and asked if anything could be done to help him. Without his parents' permission laser was used on all the acu-points. The boy was told that if he wanted any further treatment, he would have to take his parents' consent. The next morning his mother rang us up. We thought for a moment that we were about to receive a lot of criticism for treating a child without his parents' permission, but were relieved and happy to hear her say that the previous night had been the first in ten years that the boy had slept without waking up with an asthma attack. The boy was treated with laser therapy for four weeks, after which he was completely free of asthma.

Mohan Dastur, male, 66 years. My experiences in the treatment of bronchial asthma with acupuncture will be incomplete if we do not mention here a very challenging case. This patient was a senior doctor who had developed severe bronchitis. This was accompanied by acute bouts of dry cough and wheezing. He had a low grade temperature. He had been on strong antibiotics and bronchodilator drugs for the past fifteen days, but his condition had not improved at all. He was depressed and exhausted with his problem and was contemplating suicide.

Acu-points were needled for removing the excess sputum which had collected in his bronchioles and was not coming out. Immediately after the first sitting, he brought out a large quantity of mucoid sputum. We stopped all his antibiotics and bronchodilators and gave him regular acupuncture therapy for fifteen days, after which he was fully cured. He is now really convinced of the miraculous powers of acupuncture.

Chronic Sinusitis. This is a common ailment which is characterized by headache and tenderness over the sinus, which occurs when the sinuses get blocked and eventually infected. There may be fever, suggesting an infection in the sinuses. The nasal mucosa is red, and a yellow and green purulent discharge may also be present.

The patient generally complains of nasal obstruction, a purulent nasal discharge with a foul odour, loss or weakened sense of smell, and general symptoms like headache and insomnia. Western therapy includes antibiotics for infection control, steam inhalation, and nasal drops.

Acupuncture therapy recommends an anti-inflammatory action and shrinks the lining of the nose. It reduces the swelling and helps in draining out the phlegm deposited in the sinuses. Sonopuncture is given over the sinuses with a small sound head and also over painful areas.

Sanjay Sinha, male, 27 years. This young man contacted us with complaints of severe headache and swelling over the face, along with persistent nasal blockage and a feeling of phlegm falling at the back of his throat all twenty-four hours of the day. He also had symptoms of recurrent sneezing, a watery nasal discharge, and itching of the eyes and nose (allergic rhinitis) associated with sinusitis. This problem had persisted for over ten years in spite of regular treatment. The patient had started greying prematurely. He had had an antral (in the bone) puncture done to drain out the sinuses, but had later developed the symptoms all over again.

Acupuncture therapy was given to him for a period of two months, during which the patient's symptoms disappeared.

An X-ray of the sinuses was done after completion of the therapy and it showed that the sinuses were now clear. He has been having a check-up for the past three years with no recurrence of symptoms.

Ravi Mathur, male, 20 years. This youngster had been suffering from continuous sneezing and nasal discharge, severe headache, cough, and a sore throat for five years. He used to sit in his shop where there was a lot of dust; this was the cause of his problem. Examination revealed acute tenderness over the frontal and maxillary sinuses.

Acupuncture therapy was given to him regularly for twenty days and then gradually withdrawn. A total of thirty sittings were given and all his symptoms subsided. He was also given auto-immunization therapy once every week for a total of ten times and this helped him in overcoming the allergy to dust. Now he is able to sit in the same surroundings of his shop as before, but without any symptoms of sneezing or a running nose.

Disorders of the Gastro-Intestinal System

Some of the common problems afflicting the gastro-intestinal system are chronic gastritis, peptic ulcers, irritable bowel syndrome (IBS), and constipation.

Chronic Gastritis and Peptic Ulcer. Chronic gastritis is a condition which is caused by overproduction of gastric juices. It generally follows an acute attack of gastritis. Usually the symptoms are distress or pain in the upper abdomen, loss of appetite, and abdominal distension. The patient feels a heavy oppression in the stomach area with nausea. Occasionally there can be a severe pain under the chest and the attack can last from several minutes to several hours. Generally gastritis occurs due to overindulgence in spicy, fried foods and tea, coffee, and alcohol.

Peptic ulcer is a condition which can often be caused by emotional disturbances. Frequent use of painkillers can also lead to a peptic ulcer. Physiologically it results from an inability of localized areas of the gastro-duodenal mucosa to withstand the digestive action of the gastric content of the pepsin enzyme. A patient suffering from a peptic ulcer complains of a cramp-like sensation in the epigastrium. This pain occurs in definite relationship to eating. A pain which occurs immediately on eating food suggests a gastric ulcer, and distress or pain occurring after 2-3 hours suggests a duodenal ulcer. Nausea and vomiting may also occur. Physical examination reveals tenderness in the epigastrium. Pain on the left side of the abdomen suggests a gastric ulcer, and on the right side, a duodenal ulcer. A barium meal examination confirms the diagnosis.

In Western medicine, the treatment of chronic gastritis and peptic ulcer is at best, palliative. The patient gets only symptomatic improvement.

R.S. Ahluwalia, male, 50 years. For 6-7 years he had been suffering from chronic gastritis with a feeling of burning and pain in the mid-epigastrium. Regular intake of antacids was required to keep him symptom-free.

Acupuncture was given to him for ten sittings. This was followed by inserting a *catgut* at an acupuncture point in the middle of the abdomen. This *catgut* provided the effect of continuous stimulation to the acupuncture point and dissolved within four weeks.

All the symptoms of gastritis subsided and the patient did not require any more medicines. He did require *catgut embedding* again after a gap of two years, but responded to it immediately and was able to eat his normal diet without any restrictions.

Mahesh Goenka, male, 32 years. Mahesh Goenka was suffering from an acute gastric ulcer when he consulted us six years ago. He had been abroad for treatment, but the drugs gave him only symptomatic and temporary relief. He complained of pain in the mid-epigastric region, along with burning, nausea, and vomiting. He was advised very strict diet control to avoid hyperacidity.

Acupuncture was started and gradually the medicines prescribed were withdrawn. He was totally asymptomatic after twenty sittings. He was given three courses of twenty sittings each and a complete cure was achieved. He is happy now that he can enjoy eating spicy food and raw chillies which he is fond of. There has been no relapse of symptoms for over five years.

Irritable Bowel Syndrome. This is a very common, chronic, and obstinate condition troubling both the patient and the doctor. Treatment with Western medicine is not yet satisfactory. The patient complains of a dull abdominal pain which is accompanied by loose stools about 3-4 times per day. Occasionally, the patient may complain of constipation. It has been found that psychological disturbances affect the bowel movements a great deal.

Acupuncture is combined with moxibustion and cupping over the abdomen in this condition and the results are quite gratifying. Acupuncture stimulation neutralises the basic abnormal electric rhythm in the colon.

Rohit Sinha, male, 32 years. Rohit Sinha came to us with complaints of a chronic irritable bowel problem that he had been suffering from for the past five years. He used to experience an extreme fullness of the abdomen after meals, nausea, abdominal distension, diarrhoea, and occasional constipation. Whenever he ate food outside home, he got loose stools. He had tried allopathic, ayurvedic, and homoeopathic treatment but without success.

Acupuncture was started and within ten sittings, his stool started to get formed. It was no longer semi-solid or loose as it used to be. The foul smell disappeared and there was no mucus. He started eating outside and did not get any abdominal cramps or recurrent bowel movements. Moxibustion was given at specific acupuncture points on the abdomen and a total course of twenty sittings was given. He has been totally asymptomatic after the therapy and has a normal bowel movement.

This gentleman also suffered concurrently from chronic sinusitis and chronic cervical spondylitis. Both these problems were also cured with acupuncture and he is now a big fan of acupuncture therapy.

Chronic Constipation. In chronic constipation the patient suffers from infrequent defecation with a passage of dry and hard faecal matter; there is a sensation of fullness in the abdomen and sluggish movement of the bowels. A healthy person moves his bowels once or twice daily. Lack of bowel movement and a daily diminishing quantity of faeces are signs of constipation. In chronic conditions, the patient experiences some heaviness and discomfort in the abdomen. There is a lack of appetite as well as eructation. In severe conditions, the patient does not respond even to a strong purgative. Lumps of faeces can be felt by palpation of the abdomen. If the faeces remain in the abdomen for too long, the patient develops intestinal ulcers. If the faeces remain in the rectum for too long, piles will result.

Acupuncture therapy with electrical stimulation of acupuncture points and moxibustion is used to treat this condition. It helps to improve the motility of the large intestine and get regular bowel movements. However, organic causes like fissures, cancer of the rectum or colon, and rectal strictures should be ruled out first.

A high roughage diet, plenty of water, exercise, avoidance of suppression of the defecatory urge, and avoiding regular use of laxatives is advised.

Mohit Bajpai, male, 33 years. A patient of chronic constipation for twenty years, Mohit Bajpai always complained of incomplete evacuation with a feeling of heaviness which used to persist throughout the day. Even in the morning, after getting up, he would not feel any bowel movements for at least 1-2 hours. This made him very uncomfortable. After several sittings, his bowel movement became regular and he began to experience complete evacuation. This eased his stress considerably and made his life better.

Menstrual Disorders

Menstrual disorders are a common complaint amongst women. These can be due to stress or hormonal imbalances. They include irregularity of the menstrual cycle, excessive or scanty bleeding, prolonged or shortened course of menstruation, and the colour of the blood being too dark or too light.

Acupuncture is extremely effective in treating all

types of menstrual disorders such as menorrhagia, metrorrhagia, oligomenorrhea, irregular menses, dysmenorrhea, and amenorrhoea.

Vimla Jain, female, 31 years. Suffering from irregular menses for ten years, she used to get her periods after every 3-4 months. The bleeding would be quite heavy and would last for ten days, often accompanied by severe pain in the lower back and abdomen. She was treated by a leading gynaecologist, but there was no change. As a last resort, she was put on hormone therapy and started to gain weight. This made her extremely upset.

Acupuncture was started in her case on the first day of her menses and continued every day for thirty days. Her next cycle started on the same date as the previous cycle, and this time the bleeding was normal and lasted for only four days.

During the next month, she was given alternate-day therapy and she had her menses on time. During the third month, twice-a-week sittings were given and a normal flow with painless menses was experienced. In the fourth month the acupuncture treatment was reduced to a once-a-week schedule, and her periods remained on schedule. For the past one year, she has been having regular cycles with no excessive bleeding, and each cycle lasts for the normal 4-5 days. All her medication was withdrawn at the start of the acupuncture treatment and she even lost five kg of weight.

Skin Diseases

Psoriasis, infantile and chronic eczema, urticaria, vitiligo, and acne are common skin problems which affect many people.

Psoriasis. This is a non-infectious disease of the skin which is characterized by irregularly shaped, slightly raised red patches with a scaly surface. Elbows, knees, and the scalp are the areas more likely to be affected. However, in chronic cases, a patient may have psoriatic patches all over his body. It is basically an autoimmune disorder and if treatment is carried out for a prolonged period, there will be noticeable improvement.

Ms Shaila, female, 15 years. Ms Shaila came to us with a history of psoriasis for the past four years. She had generalized patches all over her body, along with severe itching and stiffness in these patches. She had tried various types of medication but had obtained no relief.

Acupuncture therapy was given to her for a period of six months. The symptomatic improvement started just after ten sittings, in that the itching and stiffness disappeared, and the scales started to fall. She was fully cured at the end of six months and has had no relapse in a follow-up period of four years.

Eczema. Eczema is an inflammation of the skin. It may be in the form of an erythema* when the skin is angry red, or there may be an eruption of pustules, blebs, and crusts. There are always scales: in some cases they are dry while others are 'weeping wet'. Eczema may affect one part of the body such as the leg, or it may affect symmetrical parts like the head and face, both hands or feet, or the whole body.

There are two types of eczema: *infantile* and *chronic*. Some cases are of occupational origin: from contact with detergents, organic solvents, chemicals, and other sensitizing materials; others are caused by the patient being allergic

* Superficial reddening of the skin, usually in patches.

to certain foods, or being affected by a systemic disease like diabetes, or due to emotional disturbances.

Western medical treatment includes topical steroid creams, oral antibiotics, and oral steroids.

Acupuncture has a definitive role to play in the treatment of this condition. Specific anti-allergic and immune-enhancing points are treated to build up body resistance and achieve a cure.

Smita Garg, female, 15 years. This girl had been suffering from severe infantile eczema, since childhood. She came to us in March, 1998 with a history of infantile eczema, manifesting itself with widespread discharging lesions over the face, elbows, hands, forearms, neck, ears, upper back, abdomen, and both legs. She used to get severe and intense itching which would not allow her to sleep at all. Her skin had started thickening and her complexion had gone darker.

She had had regular treatment since childhood from the top skin specialists and used all types of topical steroid ointments and oral medication, but to no avail.

Acupuncture was started on her from March 30, 1998, and she was asked to stop all topical and oral medicine. There was a good initial improvement and her itching reduced. Acupuncture was combined with soft laser therapy wherein the discharging lesions are exposed to infra-red lasers of 40 mw power for a duration of 1-2 minutes each.

The clinical improvement in this patient within four months was substantial. All her lesions cleared up. There was no further itching or discharge anywhere in the body. Her skin texture is now perfectly smooth and her complexion has started getting fairer.

Suman Deshpande, female, 44 years. This lady had been suffering from severe eczematous weeping lesions on her hands and legs for three years. She got terrible itching in the lesions, which used to then bleed with a watery discharge. Many topical creams and antihistamine tablets had been tried but to no avail.

Within ten days of starting acupuncture therapy, the lesions on her hands and legs started drying up. The itching reduced considerably and she began to feel much better. After three months of therapy, the lesions had healed completely and her skin texture returned to normal. There has been no relapse of the problem since.

Urticaria. Urticaria is an allergic problem, in which a patient develops wheals* marked with intolerable itching. There are numerous causes such as allergy to food, drugs, and worm infestation. The onset is quite abrupt with plaques of varying sizes and intense itching. Most of the acute cases are caused by ingestion of foods like eggs, milk, tomatoes, and chocolates. Another common cause is ingestion of drugs such as penicillin, belladonna, and salicylates. Frequent attacks of urticaria makes it a chronic disease.

Western medicine offers only symptomatic relief in the form of antihistaminic drugs, oral steroids, and topical antipruritic preparations.

Radha Kapoor, female, 25 years. Radha Kapoor had been suffering from recurrent episodes of urticaria for three years. She had tried different therapies but none had cured her problem. Acupuncture treatment was started on her on the same day that an acute attack of urticaria

---

* A localized area of edema on the body surface, often with severe itching; it is the typical lesion of urticaria.

occurred. Within forty-five minutes of needling, the itching totally subsided and the patches reduced in height. A complete course of twenty sittings was given to her and she has not had any relapse for the last one year.

Vitiligo. This is a condition in which patches of depigmentation are seen. The cause of vitiligo is largely unknown though it may be hereditary in about thirty per cent of cases. Limited to certain areas, there can also be an increase in the quantity of melanin, thus darkening those areas permanently.

Homoeopuncture has been found to produce noticeable changes in localized vitiligo, although the treatment is prolonged.

Shikha, female, 14 years. A young girl, Shikha, came to us with two patches of depigmentation over the back of her hand. These patches had been gradually increasing in size. We used the homoeopathic medicine Sepia in liquid form (strength 30) by dipping acupuncture needles into the medicine and then inserted them into the patch. About four needles were inserted into each patch. In about ten sittings small black spots had started coming out over the white patches.

However, after the next ten days, when no further black spots appeared, the strength of Sepia was increased to 200. Within ten sittings, the general colour of the patch was dark. Tapping with a plum blossom needle was also done over both the patches and this also helped in quickening the process of melanin production.

It took approximately three months for both the patches to be completely pigmented. This is a typical example of the result achieved with homoeopuncture.

Acne. Pimples on the face, back, and shoulders generally occur during puberty. This is the most common form of all skin problems. It is caused by a genetic predisposition and activated by androgens. The skin lesions are caused by sebaceous overactivity, retention of sebum, and overgrowth of the acne bacillus in the sebum.

Western medical treatment uses acne lotions, ointments, and antibiotics, usually without any success.

Madhu Raheja, female, 18 years. Madhu Raheja started hating her face as it was full of acne. She consulted many doctors, and each prescribed a different therapy. But there was no positive response. We treated her with a helium-neon laser. Within one month her face was absolutely spotless and she never had acne after that.

Eye Disorders

Acupuncture is extremely useful in the management of eye diseases like myopia, chronic conjunctivitis, optic nerve atrophy, retinitis, glaucoma, and night-blindness.

Sjogren's Syndrome. This is an eye-related problem in which there is a combination of dryness of the eyes, dryness of the mouth, increased thirst, and joint pains.

Sudha Mallya, female, 50 years. An interesting case was of a doctor, who was suffering from Sjogren's syndrome. She had developed infection of both eyes followed by dryness, intolerance to light, irritation, redness, and flake formation in the eyes. To remedy the dryness of her eyes, she had to put in artificial tears after every fifteen minutes. After six weeks she developed dryness of the mouth and nose along with a bloody discharge from the ear. She had to use nasal drops every 2-3 hours, even at night. Joint pains started after three months and the RA (rheumatoid arthritis) factor in her blood test was positive.

At this stage acupuncture was started. Within a week, the eye and mouth dryness improved. The ear discharge, nose blockage, and joint pains improved by the second week and stopped completely by the third week. As soon as acupuncture was started the flake formation disappeared. An eye specialist checked her eyes and said that her tear formation was normal and that there was no evidence of swelling or ulcer formation in the eyes. She is now about eighty per cent better and is still under our treatment.

This disease has no treatment in allopathy or any other system of medicine.

Optic Atrophy. This is a condition in which there is a wasting away or near total disuse of the eyes.

Krishna Khattar, female, 57 years. She came for the first time on January 15, 1998, with complaints of complete loss of vision in both eyes. She was only able to make out hand movements, but was unable to count the fingers. Her history revealed that she had been suffering from recurrent fever with chills from December, 1996. The fever was associated with loss of appetite and loss of weight. She was investigated for the same. A chest X-ray showed prominence of the left hilum which was most likely due to enlarged left hilar lymph nodes.

Krishna Khattar's case was diagnosed as pulmonary tuberculosis and she was put on ATT (Anti Tubercular Therapy) from May 3, 1997. She started noticing slight blurring of vision from September, 1997. This blurring worsened on October18, 1997. It was accompanied with formication* in both feet and associated tiredness. Her visual acuity at this stage was 6/36.

She was diagnosed as having acute Ethambutol toxicity and her Ethambutol was stopped. She was treated for pan uveitis** (bilateral). The VEP (Visual Evoked Potential) done at the Rajendra Prasad Ophthalmic Centre showed prolonged latency. A trial of systemic steroids was given with no improvement in vision. A perimetry (charting for any visual blind spots) done at the All India Institute of Medical Sciences (AIIMS), Delhi on November 18 showed poor fixation with poor response in both eyes. A brain MRI done on December 13 was normal. She was seen by a team of top doctors at AIIMS and then at Mohan Eye Institute, Delhi, but medication produced no improvement. Her vision steadily went on deteriorating and she was diagnosed as having developed bilateral toxic optic nerve atrophy for which there was no treatment possible. She even tried homoeopathy medicine with no response.

Acupuncture treatment was given to her initially on a daily basis for a duration of about two months. Within the first week of treatment, her vision showed such a sudden change that a woman who had not been able to move out of her room without support, was able to read the number plate of her car. Her vision gradually went on improving and the treatment was reduced to an alternate-day schedule. She was then given acupuncture only twice a week. The improvement in her vision was substantial and she regained seventy-five per cent of her vision.

---

* A sensation as of ants crawling over the skin.

** Inflammation of all the layers of both the eyes.

In order to clinically correlate the symptomatic improvement, she was referred to Dr S.N. Jha at Sir Ganga Ram Hospital, Delhi on June 11, 1998. He checked her vision and found it to be 6/18 and 6/24. He also did perimetry on this patient and found a substantial improvement as compared to the previous perimetry done at AIIMS. Even he was amazed to see such an improvement. This patient finally improved her vision by ninety-five per cent.

Psychiatric Disorders

Common psychiatric disorders are general lethargy and neurasthenia, anxiety and depression, and impotence.

General Lethargy and Neurasthenia. This is a functional disturbance of the central nervous system caused by a temporary imbalance of higher central activity (in the frontal lobe of the brain) induced by mental factors. It occurs mainly in young and middle-aged people. Neurasthenia can be caused by excessive school work during adolescence, prolonged exertion of the brain, mental worries, overindulgence in sex, alcohol, smoking, or overwork.

The key symptoms include fatigue, weakness, headache, sweating, excessive urination, tinnitus or ringing in the ears, dizziness, fear, easy exhaustion upon slight effort, lack of concentration, irritability, poor memory, poor sleep, and numerous aches and pains.

If the patient complains of the above symptoms, but no organic pathologic changes are found on physical examination, then neurasthenia can be diagnosed.

This is becoming a more common problem in middle-aged men and women who are working and are under excessive mental stress and strain.

K.C. Rathore, male, 35 years. A company executive who was doing quite well, K.C. Rathore, in his overambitious zeal to do even better, suddenly started developing symptoms of excess fatigue, loss of memory, impotence, ringing in the ears, irritability, aches and pains all over the body, and lack of sleep. All the routine investigations were carried out and no organic or pathological changes were found. He tried many ayurvedic and homoeopathic remedies too, but to no avail.

Acupuncture treatment was given to him once daily for thirty minutes for a month, and he was able to return to his normal condition.

Anxiety and Depression. Anxiety is a common ailment which does not respond well to treatment with conventional medicine. Conventional treatment uses tranquillizers and antidepressants which cause other side-effects.

Anxiety is a manifestation of an imbalance in the various neurotransmitters in the brain. The patient is treated daily until an improvement is seen. The frequency of treatment is then reduced to twice a week until the patient has responded adequately to treatment.

Narinder Chopra, male, 52 years. For eight years, Narinder Chopra had been suffering from restlessness, excessive worrying, shallow sleep for a short duration of time, and nervous weakness. He had been treated by psychiatrists and psychologists and had been taking strong antidepressant drugs and tranquillizers for relief of his symptoms. When we examined him, we found that he was feeling very low and had no interest in his surroundings.

Acupuncture therapy was started and after twenty sittings, he started feeling more active and energetic. His sleep pattern improved considerably. We started withdrawing his drugs gradually and tapered off acupuncture to thrice a week. After a while, it was reduced to a twice-a-week schedule and the drugs were gradually totally withdrawn. By then the patient was feeling very cheerful without the need for therapy or drugs.

Impotence. Impotence is essentially an inability of the male to attain or sustain a satisfactory erection for normal coitus; or a constant failure to maintain intromission of a sufficient duration to satisfy a responsive partner. Premature ejaculation refers to a much-too-rapid achievement of climax during sexual intercourse. Psychic factors are considered to be the cause in about ninety per cent of the cases of erectile dysfunction.

B.M. Mathur, male, 47 years. B.M. Mathur had a sedentary occupation and complained of impotence of several years' duration. Investigations found no organic cause, although questioning the patient indicated that it was not purely psychological as he had never woken up with an erection. He was given acupuncture therapy along with moxibustion. Sedation was applied to certain points to reduce the anxiety associated with this problem. After five weeks of treatment, the patient reported that he was cured of the problem.

Obesity

Obesity is an abnormal accumulation of fat in the stores of adipose tissues throughout the body. The main parameters of measuring obesity are the weight and height of the individual. A suitable working rule for treatment of obesity is that the weight of the patient should be brought down to within ten per cent of the desirable weight for any given height. Obesity can lead to many diseases like diabetes, heart attacks, various types of body pains, high blood pressure, and asthmatic conditions.

The patient should first be thoroughly investigated to find out the cause of overweight. Most patients of overweight are so due to overeating. However, endocrine disorders must be ruled out before planning the treatment.

A patient is put on acupuncture therapy which helps to control the appetite and reduce the urge to eat by fifty per cent. He/she is advised a diet chart which involves taking three meals regularly with no fad diets or starvation. A set of exercises is also advised to burn fat faster.

World Health Organization (WHO) recommends that an ideal weight loss of one kg per week is sufficient, and gradual weight loss is always better so that the patient does not tend to gain back the lost weight again.

Preeti Sahni, female, 25 years. After delivering a child Preeti Sahni put on weight. Luckily the weight loss required in her case was just about five kg. She was given treatment at the ear acupuncture points twice a week with electrostimulation, and a press needle was inserted at the stomach point in both the ears. She was advised to press the needles about half an hour before each meal and in-between whenever she felt the urge to eat. This helped in controlling her hunger pangs and reduced her overall intake of food by fifty per cent. She lost five kg weight in a period of two months.

Sudha Sood, female, 41 years. A grossly overweight woman, Sudha Sood came for acupuncture therapy to reduce weight. She lost seven kg in the first month, five kg in the second month, three kg in the third month, and two kg in the fourth month. She lost a total of seventeen kg in a span of four months.

Smoking

Acupuncture is an extremely effective mode of treatment in the management of cigarette and alcohol addicts.

Ramesh Basu, male, 40 years. A captain in the navy, Ramesh Basu used to smoke about twenty cigarettes a day. Needles were applied to the acupuncture points in the ear once daily, for ten days. He felt that his urge to smoke came down drastically and he started disliking the taste of cigarettes. He reduced his intake to just five cigarettes a day. Another course of ten sittings was given and he was able to give up smoking totally.

Connie D'Souza, female, 58 years. Connie D'Souza was on a visit to India when she met us with her friend whom we were going to treat for an acute back sprain. The lady was used to smoking sixty cigarettes a day and in the words of her friend, was 'never seen without a cigarette in her mouth'! She asked us if acupuncture would stop her from smoking. She had been smoking from the age of fifteen and in the last forty-three years, had stuck to the habit. She was given acupuncture at the lung and addiction points in both the ears which were electrically stimulated for thirty minutes. After the removal of the needles, a small press needle was placed in the lung point of the right ear and the patient was instructed to press on it at least three times per day and whenever she felt the urge to smoke. Not only did she never smoke again, but about six weeks later, she rang up to tell us that after the acupuncture treatment, she felt as though she had never smoked. She said that she felt very fit and was adamant that she would never return to the domination of 'Lady Nicotine'!

13

Frequently Asked Questions

Q. *What is the meaning of the word acupuncture?*

A. Acupuncture is derived from latin words 'acus' and 'puncture', where *acus* means 'needle' and *puncture* means 'to penetrate'.

Q. *What factors determine the response of a patient to acupuncture?*

A. The response of a patient to acupuncture is dependent on the severity of the illness and the length of time the patient has suffered from it. Other important factors are the general health, constitutional type, emotional balance, diet, lifestyle, and any medication the patient has received in the past or is receiving at the time of consultation.

Q. *What factors affect the effectiveness of acupuncture treatment?*

A. Acupuncture's effectiveness depends on its ability to improve the flow of *Qi* (the life-force, vitality, or energy that makes us alive) in the body. If *Qi* is very depleted, or if its flow is blocked, progress will be slow or even non-existent. In conditions of great depletion the patient's constitution must be built up for acupuncture to have an effect. A patient's refusal to make recommended changes in diet or lifestyle may reduce the treatment's effectiveness. In a patient receiving medication from an orthodox practitioner, especially on a long-term basis, acupuncture treatment is likely to be difficult and take some time to be effective.

Q. *How quickly can acupuncture treat an illness?*

A. It is difficult to generalize about how quickly or slowly acupuncture will work. The response varies from individual to individual. Acupuncture's speed is dependent on *Qi*, so children and those with good general vitality often respond fast, but older people and those with depleted *Qi*'s may expect slower results. The duration of treatment is decided by the duration of illness. The less chronic an illness, lesser are the number of sittings required.

Q. *Does acupuncture cure a problem or provide temporary relief?*

A. Acupuncture cures many diseases like bronchial asthma, cervical spondylitis, low backache, acne, frozen shoulder, etc. However, in some diseases like rheumatoid arthritis, anxiety neurosis, prolapsed disc, etc., it provides symptomatic relief and the patient has to take treatment at regular intervals to achieve improvement.

Q. *It is effective as a single mode of treatment or in conjunction with others?*

A. It is generally effective as a single mode of treatment.

Q. *Does it reduce/increase/hamper the effects of other simultaneous treatments?*

A. It does not alter the effect of any other simultaneous treatment.

Q. *Has acupuncture been given formal scientific recognition?*

A. Yes, it has been given scientific recognition by the WHO and in many other countries like Sri Lanka, Australia, UK, and USA the government have acupuncture councils. In India presently the recognition of acupuncture is under the active consideration of the government. The West Bengal government has already recognized acupuncture in their state. Research projects on acupuncture have been financed by the Indian Council of Medical Research (ICMR) and the Centre for Scientific and Industrial Research (CSIR) at the Ranjit Memorial Acupuncture Hospital, Howrah, West Bengal.

Q. *What is the cost of acupuncture treatment?*

A. The cost of acupuncture treatment varies from doctor to doctor and city to city. A single sitting in Delhi or Mumbai may cost Rs 150 upwards (at 1999 prices).

Q. *Which painful conditions can be treated by acupuncture?*

A. Acupuncture can treat any pain of the body, ranging from headache, neck pain, low back pain, sciatica, joint pains, ankle pains — even cancer pains.

Q. *Can it treat any other condition besides pain?*

A. Yes, it can treat a large number of diseases like polio, paralysis, asthma, sinusitis, eczema, deafness, constipation, menstrual problems, hyperacidity, hypertension, psoriasis, facial paralysis, vertigo, laryngitis, obesity, acne, optic atrophy, chronic bronchitis, and all chronic diseases.

Q. *Does acupuncture have any side-effects?*

A. Acupuncture does not have any side or after effects.

Q. *Is the insertion of needles painful?*

A. Prior to their first treatment, many people do not believe that acupuncture can be painless. Different sensations such as warmth or pressure may be felt, but the energetic sensation differs from pain. People often comment that the feeling is unfamiliar but pleasant and relaxing. Acupuncture needles are very fine, about the size of a thick hair. They are solid and nothing is injected through them. Over the centuries, refined needle insertion techniques have been developed which enable the skilled acupuncturist to place a needle with little or no pain.

Q. *Is there any bleeding with needles?*

A. There is no bleeding with acupuncture needles.

Q. *How often are the needles used in acupuncture changed?*

A. Most practitioners will use disposable needles if requested, although all registered acupuncturists are required to carry out stringent sterilization procedures so this is not strictly necessary.

Q. *What treatments are available for patients who are apprehensive of needles?*

A. A number of needleless techniques such as Transcutaneous Electro-Acupuncture, Laser Acupuncture, Sonopuncture, and Stipuncture are available for patients who are apprehensive of needles.

Q. *What is the benefit of electrical stimulation?*

A. Electrical stimulation reduces the time required per treatment and is very useful in treating acute conditions.

It is more reliable, less tiring, and more acceptable to the patient.

Q. *What is meant by preventive acupuncture?*

A. Acupuncture can spot the start of trouble — before the acute phase begins — by identifying the tendencies that could develop into illness. Treatment at this stage ensures the prevention of the illness. This is called preventive acupuncture.

Q. *What role can acupuncture play in childbirth?*

A. Acupuncture has two main effects in childbirth: it can reduce pain; and it can stimulate the contractions of the uterus, which help to ensure a healthy delivery. Reduction of pain without the use of drugs is of special benefit, especially to the unborn child.

Q. *Does acupuncture offer any hope to AIDS patients?*

A. Acupuncture is being increasingly used in the treatment of AIDS, but this being a recent phenomenon it is difficult to assess the benefits. In the early stages, acupuncture can be very helpful to re-activate the immune system, and at all stages can help to deal with the wide range of symptoms which tend to manifest.

Q. *Can acupuncture be used to quit smoking?*

A. Acupuncture treatment helps to reduce or even give up smoking. It makes the system more sensitive to toxins, and may make a patient feel that smoking is repellant. The patient must be committed to stopping smoking as acupuncture treatment can only help the nicotine addict — it is not a miracle cure.

Q. *Is acupuncture helpful in sleeping problems?*

A. It is important to understand that very often sleeping problems are a result of stress. If sleeping pills have been prescribed, it is essential that they are not continued to a point at which dependence, whether psychological or physical can occur. Should the patient feel unable to cope without sleeping pills, acupuncture can play a positive role by helping reduce the drug, while assisting in regulating the patient's sleeping pattern. Bringing the sleeping pattern to normal may take 4-6 weeks and the patient should be able to sleep without the aid of drugs.

Q. *Is acupuncture effective in emotional problems?*

A. The Chinese philosophy of health does not distinguish between physical and mental problems: both are treated at the same time, and are seen as different manifestations of one pattern of disharmony. Emotional imbalances, if untreated, may eventually result in physical symptoms, and are considered by the Chinese to be one of the major causes of disease. These emotional imbalances are treated by rebalancing, removing blockages, and restoring the natural flow of energy, and not by suppressing symptoms with potentially addictive medicines.

Q. *What are the limitations of acupuncture?*

A. Apart from limitations in the practitioner's knowledge and skill, and in a patient's willingness to heed advice, the most significant practical restriction is the need for a practitioner to be present in order for treatment to be given. In China this problem is tackled by prescribing herbal remedies to be taken between consultations.

An 'emergency' patient needing life-saving resuscitation or surgery or suffering from a serious infection, any life-threatening condition, or a mechanical problem must be immediately directed to the nearest hospital. In such conditions acupuncture would normally be a useful supplement in improving the final outcome of the sickness, and curing the residual/chronic component of the sickness.

Bibliography

Traditional Chinese Medicine

Anonymous. *An Outline of Chinese Acupuncture.* Peiking: The Academy of Traditional Chinese Medicine.

Kaptchuk, T.J. *Chinese Medicine: The Web Has No Weaver.* London: (Rider) Hutchinson Publishing Group Ltd., 1983.

Macdonald, A. *Acupuncture: From Ancient Art to Modern Medicine.* London: George Allen and Unwin, 1984.

Needham, J., L. Gwei-Djen. *Celestial Lancets: A History and Rationale of Acupuncture and Moxa.* Cambridge: Cambridge University Press, 1980.

Scientific Acupuncture

Mann, K.F. *The Treatment of Disease by Acupuncture.* 3rd ed. London: Heinemann Books, 1980.

Melzack, R., P.D. Wall. *The Challenge of Pain.* Harmondsworth: Penguin Books, 1982.

Travell, J.G., D.G. Simons. *Myofascial Pain and Dysfunction: The Trigger Point Manual.* Baltimore/ London: Williams and Wilkins.

Scheindeman, Dr Ian. *Medical Acupuncture.* 1st ed. Hong Kong: National Library of Australia, 1988.

Stux, Dr G., B. Pomeranz. *Basics of Acupuncture.* 2nd ed. Heidelberg, Germany: Springer Verlag, 1991.

Nightingale, Dr Michael. *Healing Power of Acupuncture.* 1st ed. Great Britain: Javelin Books, 1986.

Kenyon, Dr Julian. *Modern Techniques of Acupuncture.* 2nd ed. Great Britain: Thorsons Publishing Group, 1986.

Seng, Dr Andrew Tiong. *Innovative Acupuncture.* 1st ed. Kuala Lumpur: A and T Health Care Distribution, 1993.

Woo, Dr Park Jae. *Guide to Hand and Foot Acupuncture.* 1st ed. Korea: Ohaeng Publishing Company, 1993.

Kapur, Dr Raman. *Soft Lasers in Medical Practice.* 1st ed. New Delhi: Jaypee Brothers Medical Publishers, 1997.

Glossary

Acuity. Clarity or clearness, especially of vision.

Adipose tissues. Fatty connective tissues.

Amenorrhea. An abnormal absence of menstruation.

Androgens. Substances capable of developing and maintaining certain male sexual characteristics.

Ankylosed. Abnormal stiffening and immobility of a joint due to fusion of bones.

Anorexia. Lack or loss of appetite for food.

Antipruritic. That which relieves itching.

Arthropathy. A disease of the joints.

Autoclave. A strong vessel used for chemical reactions at high pressures and temperatures.

Autoimmune disorder. One caused by antibodies produced against substances naturally present in the body.

Blebs. Small blisters on the skin.

Bursa. A fluid-filled sac or sac-like cavity especially one countering friction at a joint.

Bursitis. Inflammation of a bursa, typically one in a shoulder joint.

Calcaneus. The bone forming the heel.

Calculi. A stone or concentration of minerals formed within the body.

Catgut. A material made of the twisted intestines of the sheep, horse, or ass and used for surgical sutures.

CAT scan. Computerized Transverse Axial Temography. A method of X-ray localization in which a thin beam of X-rays scans the body in a series of planes and results are displayed on a screen. It is used for studying the cross-section of various internal organs (e.g. brain, spine, liver, abdomen, etc.).

Centrifugal. A gradually widening circular movement which moves away from the centre.

Centripetal. Moving towards the centre.

Cervicitis. Inflammation of the cervix uteri.

Cyanosis. A bluish discolouration of skin and mucous membranes due to excessive concentration of reduced haemoglobin in the blood.

Dysmenorrhea. Painful menstruation.

ECG. Electrocardiogram. A graphic tracing of the variations in electrical potential caused by the excitation of the heart muscle and detected at the body surface.

Embolism. The obstruction of an artery by a blood clot or an air-bubble.

Encephalins. These are compounds that occur in the brain and have pain-relieving properties similar to those of morphine.

Encephalitis. Inflammation of the brain.

Endorphins. These are compounds that occur in the brain and have pain-relieving properties similar to those of morphine.

Epigastrium. The part of the abdomen immediately over the stomach.

ESR. Erythrocyte Sedimentation Rate. It is measured by a ESR meter which finds the degree of arousal of the sympathetic nervous system by measuring the skin resistance.

Fibromyalgia. Painful inflammation of fibres and muscles.

Fibrositis. Painful inflammation of fibrous connective tissue.

Gamma globulin. Antibodies which increase immunity.

Ganglion. A knot, or knotlike mass of nerves.

Gluteai. Muscles of the buttock region.

Glycoprotein. Any of a group of compounds consisting of a protein combined with a carbohydrate.

Herpes zoster. Inflammatory disease of the nerve roots and nerves, characterized by small vesicles and pain.

Hilum. A depression or pit on an organ, giving entrance and exit to vessels and nerves.

Homoeostatis. Balancing the body energy.

Hyperesthesia. An excessive physical sensitivity, especially of the skin.

Infarct. A small localised area of dead tissue caused by an inadequate blood supply.

Lithotomy. Incision of a duct or organ for removal of calculi.

Menorrhalgia. Abnormally heavy bleeding at menstruation.

Metrorrhagia. Abnormal bleeding from the womb.

MRI. Magnetic Resonance Imaging.

Oligomenorrhea. Abnormal scanty menstruation.

Periosteum. A specialised connective tissue, covering all bones and possessing bone-forming potential.

Plantar. Of or relating to the sole of the foot.

Point detector. A device to find the exact location of acupuncture points.

Sacroiliac joints. Joints of the lower sacrum.

Sacrum. A triangular bone formed from fused vertebrae and situated between the two hip-bones of the pelvis.

Sebum. The oily secretion of the sebaceous glands.

Sedation. Reduce (in excess disease).

Shiatsu. A therapy of Japanese origin, in which pressure is applied with the thumbs and palms to certain points in the body.

Stagnation. Blockage of energy flow.

Sternomastoid. Pertaining to the sternum and mastoid process (a conical prominence on the temporal bone behind the ear, to which muscles are attached).

Synovial membrane. A dense membrane of connective tissue secreting a fluid which lubricates joints and tendons.

Systolic. The contraction of the heart when blood is pumped into the arteries.

Tachycardia. An abnormally rapid heart rate.

Thrombosis. The coagulation of the blood in a blood vessel or organ.

Tonifying. Increase (in deficiency disease).

Traction. A sustained pulling on a limb, muscle, etc., by means of pulleys, weights etc.

Appendix

Addresses of Hospitals in India Offering Acupuncture Treatment

- Oil India Limited Hospital
  Duliajan, Assam.
- All India Institute of Medical Sciences (AIIMS)
  Ansari Nagar
  New Delhi-110 029.
- Batra Hospital and Medical Research Centre
  1, Tughlakabad Institutional Area
  Mehrauli-Badarpur Road
  New Delhi-110 062.
- Guru Teg Bahadur Hospital
  Shahdara,
  Delhi-110 095.
- Maulana Azad Medical College
  Bahadur Shah Zafar Marg
  New Delhi-110 002.
- Ram Manohar Lohia Hospital
  Baba Kharak Singh Marg
  New Delhi-110 001.
- Safdarjung Hospital
  New Delhi-110 029.
- Sanjay Gandhi Memorial Hospital
  New Delhi.
- Sir Ganga Ram Hospital
  Ganga Ram Hospital Marg
  Rajinder Nagar
  New Delhi-110 060.

- Post-graduate Institute of Medical Education and Research
Chandigarh.
- NTPC Hospital
Korba, Madhya Pradesh.
- Tata Memorial Hospital
Mumbai, Maharashtra.
- Indian Acupuncture Research Institute
C Scheme, Jaipur, Rajathan.
- G.B. Hospital
Agartala, Tripura.
- B.K. Basu Memorial Research Institute of Acupuncture
S.N.P. Hospital
Calcutta-700 020,
West Bengal.
- Sambhunath Pandit Hospital
Calcutta, West Bengal.
- Chittaranjan Cancer Hospital
Calcutta, West Bengal.
- N.C.C.H. Medical College and Hospital, Howrah,
West Bengal.
- University College of Science
Calcutta, West Bengal.
- Dr Kotnis Memorial Hospital
Calcutta, West Bengal.
- Medical College
Acupuncture Clinic
Calcutta, West Bengal.
- R. Ahmed Dental College
Acupuncture Clinic
Calcutta, West Bengal.
- Ranjit Memorial
Acupuncture Hospital
Howrah, West Bengal.
- R.G. Kar Medical College
Acupuncture Clinic
Calcutta, West Bengal.